Supervision for Early Years Workers

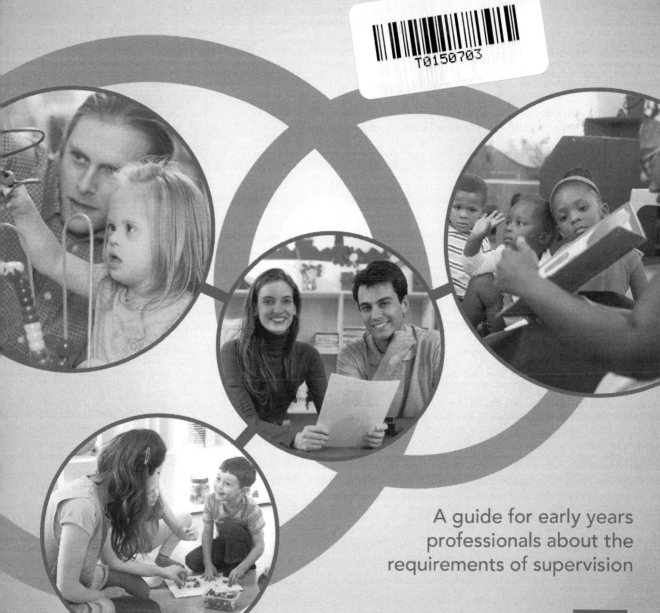

A guide for early years
professionals about the
requirements of supervision

Pavilion

Penny Sturt and Jane Wonnacott

Supervision for Early Years Workers
A guide for early years professionals about the requirements of supervision

© Penny Sturt and Jane Wonnacott, 2016

The authors have asserted their rights in accordance with the Copyright, Designs and Patents Act (1988) to be identified as the authors of this work.

Published by:
Pavilion Publishing and Media Ltd
Rayford House
School Road
Hove
East Sussex
BN3 5HX
Tel: 01273 434 943
Fax: 01273 227 308
Email: info@pavpub.com

Published 2016

A catalogue record for this book is available from the British Library.

PRINT ISBN: 978-1-910366-84-4
EPUB ISBN: 978-1-910366-85-1
EPDF ISBN: 978-1-910366-86-8
MOBI ISBN: 978-1-910366-87-5

Pavilion is the leading training and development provider and publisher in the health, social care and allied fields, providing a range of innovative training solutions underpinned by sound research and professional values. We aim to put our customers first, through excellent customer service and value.

Authors: Penny Sturt and Jane Wonnacott
Production editor: Ruth Chalmers, Pavilion Publishing and Media Ltd
Cover design: Emma Dawe, Pavilion Publishing and Media Ltd
Page layout and typesetting: Emma Dawe, Pavilion Publishing and Media Ltd
Printing: CMP Digital Print Solutions

Contents

Penny Sturt is an independent trainer, consultant and registered social worker. Following her advanced social work training which developed her interest in supervision, Penny has been delivering supervision training as an associate with In-Trac Training and Consultancy Ltd. Penny has used her knowledge, skills and experience in supervision to work with early years providers in adapting supervision for early years settings. Penny has a keen interest in supporting practitioners to deliver high quality, compassionate and stimulating care to young children and sees supervision as an effective method to do this. She is also a custodial trustee and a safeguarding adviser to early years providers.

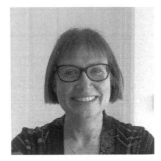

Jane Wonnacott is director of professional practice at In-Trac Training and Consultancy Ltd. She qualified as a social worker in 1979 and for the past 20 years has been working as an independent trainer and consultant. In this role she has worked with numerous statutory and voluntary organisations developing and delivering training as well as working on other projects including practice audits, policy development and serious case reviews. Jane has a long-standing interest in supervision and has developed and delivered supervision training courses both in the UK and abroad. She co-wrote, with Tony Morrison, the Children's Workforce Development Council's guide and training programme for the supervisors of social workers in the first three years of their professional development. Since Tony's death in 2010, In-Trac have continued to develop these training materials and from 2009–2014 trained over 10,000 supervisors working within health and social care. Jane is also author of *Mastering Social Work Supervision* (2012), published by Jessica Kingsley Publishers.

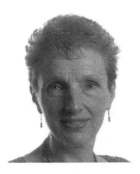

Introduction to the guide

This guide is designed to support early years providers in the delivery of effective staff supervision. Since 2012 the Early Years Foundation Stage (EYFS) has recognised the importance of supervision and the current framework (Department for Education, 2014) states that:

> *'Providers must put appropriate arrangements in place for the supervision of staff who have contact with children and families. Effective supervision provides support, coaching and training for the practitioner and promotes the interests of children.*
>
> *Supervision should foster a culture of mutual support, teamwork, and continuous improvement which encourages the confidential discussion of sensitive issues.'*
> (Department for Education, 2014, para 3.21)

Although this sets out the framework of expectations in relation to supervision, there are still many differing ideas as to what good supervision looks like in practice and how this can be provided by a busy early years manager.

This guide aims to support the delivery of supervision in practice by answering three fundamental questions:

- Why is supervision so important?
- What are the core components of supervision?
- How can a supervisor and supervisee work together to make supervision effective?

Why is supervision so important?

Practitioners are the most important resource for any early years provider and the strength of the practitioners will make a significant difference to the success of the provision and outcomes for the children receiving the service. Providing effective supervision is fundamental to nurturing and developing practitioners so that they can do the best possible job.

We want practitioners to develop good professional relationships with children where they can provide support but also challenge them to develop. Similarly parents often need support but from time to time we may need to challenge them to think differently about the care they give to their child. This mixture of support and challenge needs to be modelled in relationships between practitioners and their managers, and supervision provides the ideal setting for this to happen. Achieving this balance is explored further in Chapter 4.

Sometimes practitioners will struggle, or you may be concerned about the quality of their work. If supervision is working well it will give you an opportunity to deal with any concerns about practice early on and support them in improving their practice. This is explored further in Chapter 2.

It goes without saying that practitioners in early years settings work with people. Any practitioner who works with people, of whatever age, is likely to experience immense rewards but also challenges and a mixture of emotions. Keeping a focus on the needs of the child and delivering high quality care will be the absolute priority of all early years providers but in order to achieve this, the needs of the practitioners delivering this care also need to be addressed. Working positively with emotions in supervision is explored further in Chapter 3.

Good supervision is also crucial to good safeguarding practice and provides the opportunity to focus on any concerns that may indicate a child's well-being is compromised either at home or within the setting itself. This is explored in Chapter 1.

What are the core components of supervision?

Sometimes supervision is confused with other management activities such as performance appraisal. While there are links between the two and supervision will feed into appraisal, supervision is a distinct activity in its own right covering a wide range of activity designed to support the supervisee in their work.

There will be different ways of delivering supervision depending on the structure of your setting and the practitioners' skills. However, there are core elements that make up effective supervisory practice. These include:

- getting to know your supervisee – developing and maintaining a good working relationship and using and reviewing a supervision agreement as the foundation for this relationship (Chapter 4)

- providing structured opportunities for discussion which include the four key aspects of supervision – management, support, development and mediation (Chapter 1)

- providing an opportunity for practitioners to reflect on their practice – this includes understanding the link between how they feel, what they think and what they do (Chapter 3)

- providing an opportunity to learn from what has gone well in addition to mistakes and using the opportunity to 'nip in the bud' any emerging concerns about practice (Chapter 2)

- recording supervision discussions (Chapter 4).

How can a supervisor and supervisee work together to make supervision effective?

Good supervision does not just happen; it needs commitment from the provision, the supervisor and the supervisee. It is this shared commitment and the belief in the positive difference it can make to day-to-day practice that will provide the foundation for effective supervision.

When work is busy it is too easy for supervision arrangements to slip, yet this is often the time when they are most important. Having a shared understanding of what each expects from the other starts with a culture within the provision which values and prioritises supervision, backed up by a written supervision policy. Why this is important is discussed further in Chapter 6.

There are also a number of practical ideas and tools that supervisors and supervisees can use which are set out in this guide. These include:

- individual supervision agreements tailored to the needs of each supervisee (Chapter 4)

- integrating coaching skills into supervision (Chapter 4)

- using the supervision cycle to reflect on practice and plan next steps (Chapter 3)

- recording formats that capture specific case issues to be added to a child's file as well as general supervision issues relating to the supervisee (Chapter 4)

- developing a supervision policy which establishes the culture of supervision (Chapter 6)

■ an audit tool to plan the management tasks of establishing effective supervision (Chapter 6).

What is most important is that there is an ongoing dialogue between supervisors and their supervisees about what works in making supervision effective, and a joint commitment to making supervision a central and effective element of day-to-day practice.

Chapter 1: Why is supervision important and what does effective supervision look like?

Introduction

What is supervision? At its simplest, supervision is *'a professional conversation'* (Department for Education, 2015). This idea of a professional conversation has been the most helpful in clarifying what is expected by the statutory requirement to provide supervision in early years settings. Supervision describes the process by which one practitioner becomes accountable for the quality of another practitioner's work. This chapter answers why supervision is important in protecting children, its role in ensuring the early years environment is safe for children and practitioners, as well as how supervision contributes to practitioner development. This guide offers a definition of supervision and compares it with the expectations laid out in the Early Years Foundation Stage (EYFS) (Department for Education, 2014). The key components are explored in this chapter.

Throughout this guide ideas are offered that have been tried out and found useful by early years practitioners.

Why is supervision needed?

The statutory framework for the EYFS now states categorically that supervision must be provided in all early years settings (Department for Education, 2014, para. 3.19). Therefore it is important that each provision establishes a culture which includes clear expectations of supervision (more detail about how to establish such a culture is provided in Chapter 6). It's essential to remember why this requirement has come into force.

Children are vulnerable to abuse, especially those under the age of five, because of their dependency on adults for their care and survival. The child protection system is used to safeguard children within the family situation. The child protection procedures within early years settings for reporting children who workers are concerned about are well established.

Children are particularly vulnerable in group care situations (Erooga, 2012). The recent focus of attention on early years settings highlights the need for providers to establish cultures which protect children within their settings from practitioners who may pose a risk (Plymouth Safeguarding Children Board, 2010; Birmingham Safeguarding Children Board, 2012). Erooga (2012) summarises the twin purposes of policies and procedures. Firstly, they should be designed to keep people who pose a risk to children out of the setting by safer recruitment and formalised checking processes. This will not by itself remove the risk of future offending but acts as a deterrent. Secondly, he also identifies that there needs to be safe practices within the setting that create a culture of vigilance and awareness around individual practitioners. This is because there are also a group of individuals '...*who abused in organisational settings and yet appeared to have no known predisposition or motivation to abuse before taking up those posts*' (Erooga, 2012, p.3).

In short, some people appear to abuse children because the opportunity arises for them. Providers need to take steps to lessen those opportunities where children are vulnerable to such abuse by having cultures of safe practice as well as expectations that practitioners challenge each other's behaviour. The issues relating to safe practices are expanded on further in Chapter 6: Establishing a culture of supervision.

Here the focus is on these individuals. An important question for providers is how to recognise the signs about these practitioners. If a colleague is concerned about behavioural changes in a practitioner or the way they are speaking about or dealing with a particular child or groups of children, how do they report those concerns in such a way that the issues are taken seriously? In the case of the Plymouth nursery (Nursery Z), practitioners had observed changes in Vanessa George's behaviour (e.g. sharing indecent images, crude use of language), yet did not know where to raise their concerns about this (Plymouth Safeguarding Children Board, 2010; Wonnacott 2013). It is important for safe practices to be adopted by early years providers and within this context a culture that reinforces the centrality and significance of supervision becomes essential. Supervision provides a structure as well as expectations of conduct; this is the person (your supervisor) you talk to about your concerns (as a supervisee).

Supervision is part of establishing and maintaining a culture of safe practice which will safeguard children and ultimately, practitioners. Supervision works best when the reasons for it are understood by all members of the setting, including volunteers or parent helpers. Policies and procedures can be protective but they are not protective by themselves. In order to be effective, all practitioners need to understand why the policies and procedures are required and how they should contribute to a safer environment for the children by taking part in professional conversations.

Using the idea of a professional conversation helps make clear what supervision is. Early years providers sometimes describe supervision as 'one to ones', a 'chat' or team meeting. This guide explores what the differences are between a chat and supervision, why there is a need for a formal professional conversation about work and how supervision assists practitioners in thinking about what they do with children. Children in early years settings need to be safe, happy and learning; supervision is one method of providers finding out if this is the case.

Knowing what supervision is, is essential in order to provide it effectively, therefore this chapter explains what supervision means. It is also important to explore the differences between supervision, mentoring, coaching and performance appraisal, and where they may be interlinked. The definition in EYFS uses these terms without explaining what they mean. This chapter explains what each term means and gives examples so supervisors understand what they are expected to do. It is also designed to help supervisees and other practitioners understand what is meant by supervision.

From the expectations in the guide *Working Together to Safeguard Children* (Department for Education, 2015) it is clear that professionals are expected to regularly review and reflect on whether the children they care for are safe and their well-being is promoted. The expectation that children are discussed with others with similar knowledge and skills is essential to the child protection process to identify children at risk of significant harm, in order to intervene early and be effective in addressing their needs (Department for Education, 2015, para. 56). The expectations of EYFS make clear that every child is a unique person with differing needs. Early years practitioners are expected to offer consistent, high quality care to children in an environment that enables their learning (Department for Education, 2014, para. 6). Meeting children's diverse needs is a key element in being an enabling environment. Supervision of practitioners plays an important part in ensuring children's learning is effectively monitored. These discussions need to be more than 'a chat over coffee' or when setting up the room before the session starts. They require clarification about the boundaries as well as what happens as a result of the discussion. How can early years providers recognise when supervision is being done well?

This chapter provides a definition and suggestions for a structure to supervision, including how it meets these expectations. The definition being used for early years providers has been adapted from the work of Morrison (2005).

'Supervision is a process by which one practitioner is given responsibility by the provision to work with another practitioner(s) in order to meet certain organisational, professional and personal objectives which together promote the best outcomes for children. These objectives and functions are:

- *competent accountable performance (managerial function)*
- *continuing professional development (developmental / formative function)*
- *personal support (supportive / restorative function)*
- *engaging the practitioner with the provision (mediation function).'*

(Morrison, 2005)

The four functions of supervision explain why supervision is a helpful process. The following questions seek to explore these functions from the perspective of practitioners.

- Are you doing what your manager thinks they are paying you to do? Everyone works better when they know what is expected of them. That is the managerial function.

- Could you improve what you are doing if given some training/different opportunities? That is the development function.

- What support do you need? What would help you, emotionally, to do your job better? That is the support function.

- Whenever you are wearing your uniform are you behaving, and therefore representing the provision, as your manager expects you to? That is the mediation function.

Each of these four functions is discussed in greater detail over the next few pages. It is important at this stage to recognise that supervision needs to be a flexible response catering to individual needs and therefore in each supervision session the four aspects will not get equal attention every time. However, having an awareness of the need for all four functions does help supervisors maintain the boundaries around supervision and prevent it being turned into a 'chat.' 'Chatting' is a necessary social skill which builds rapport and relationships between practitioners working together. Supervision is effective when there is a trusting relationship built between supervisor and supervisee. Therefore some chat to build rapport and trust may form part of supervision. However supervision needs to move swiftly on from chatting into the purpose of supervision summarised in the four functions.

The managerial function

Early years practitioners, in order to do their best, need to be clear about what they are being asked to do, in what manner and by when. Are practitioners or volunteers doing the job they are expected to? Supervision provides the means to discuss these accountabilities, to be clear what supervisors expect from their practitioners; for example which issues should be brought to a manager's attention immediately and which can wait. As a supervisor you need to know straight away if a practitioner has serious, immediate concerns about a child's well-being, but could wait for a planned supervision session to discuss their holiday leave.

Practitioners require feedback on their performance. They need supervisors to notice what they have done well and to be offered the opportunity to reflect on things they could improve with constructive advice. Some effective supervisors jot down their observations of good practice at the time, so that they remember to praise practitioners in supervision for the examples of good work they have observed since their last formal meeting. Knowing good work is noticed may make it easier for practitioners to ask for help with tasks which feel difficult.

Thinking point

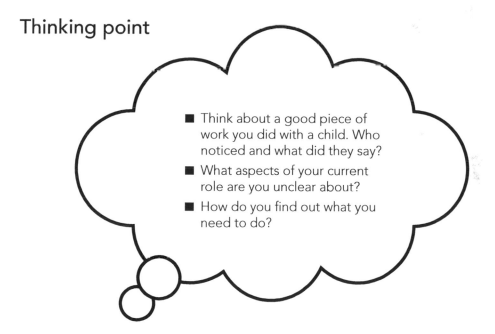

■ Think about a good piece of work you did with a child. Who noticed and what did they say?

■ What aspects of your current role are you unclear about?

■ How do you find out what you need to do?

The developmental function

Early years providers need to know that practitioners are developing their capabilities and competence. In this changing world of increasing expectations it can be challenging at times to ensure practitioners are knowledgeable, able to use their skills competently and have the requisite training for the job. An important element of supervision is to ensure practitioners keep improving their skills as the expectations of practitioners working in early years keep changing. It is the responsibility of supervisors to ensure practitioners have opportunities to keep acquiring the skills they need. Practitioners are increasingly expected to have good literacy, numeracy and computing skills, but when they entered the workforce those requirements may not have been there, so supervision needs to be a space to look for strategies to develop these competencies. For instance, perhaps there is a practitioner who has a good grasp of ways to stimulate children's intellectual curiosity and likes to find different ways of getting children to play. Is she someone to nurture and encourage into taking a role where these skills are required, such as to co-ordinate the Education, Health and Care (EHC) plans for the provision?

Supervision is also a space to reflect on the value base practitioners are using. Are they able to think about how children and parents with diverse needs use the provision? For example, how accessible is the provision for a child/parent with disabilities, or how is the 'Child's Journey' made available to a child who is visually impaired? Supervision is effective when practitioners are able to make links between their experiences and decide what will help them improve their professional development. When a supervisee notices a training course or an interest they wish to develop, the supervisor knows they are being effective.

Thinking point

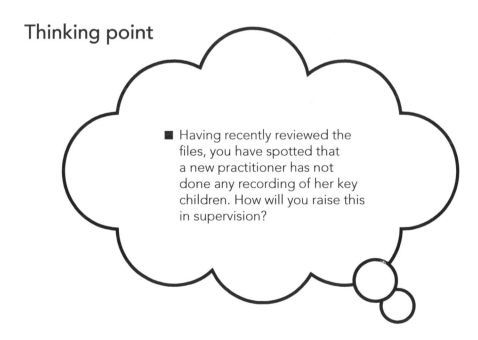

- Having recently reviewed the files, you have spotted that a new practitioner has not done any recording of her key children. How will you raise this in supervision?

The supportive function

Supervision is a vehicle for ensuring practitioners feel supported in their role. Working with children can be exhausting (as well as immensely enjoyable). Sometimes children will be distressed by events in their lives, for example a new baby, or a parent leaving. Sometimes practitioners will be finding life difficult too because of bereavement, relationship breakdown and so on. Early years practitioners need a confidential space to offload. Supervision can be that space to talk about how practitioners are feeling if their key child is very distressed or if they are sad about the events in their own life. The skill of the effective supervisor is understanding the limits of the supportive function. Emotional support is crucial to allow practitioners to perform to their optimum capabilities. However if a practitioner is so distressed it is affecting their ability to work the supervisor may need to recognise and manage this by encouraging them to consider counselling and/or managing absence.

Supervision is an opportunity to monitor the effects of the job and ensure practitioners are coping and not becoming stressed by the demands of their work. Supervision may equally be an opportunity to encourage creativity in trying new things out in an atmosphere of praise and encouragement. Supervision, if used effectively, ensures practitioners remain attuned to children's needs, are not overwhelmed by their distress and are able to take opportunities to be creative.

Thinking point

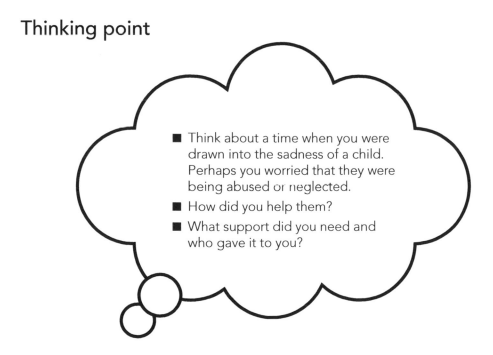

- Think about a time when you were drawn into the sadness of a child. Perhaps you worried that they were being abused or neglected.
- How did you help them?
- What support did you need and who gave it to you?

The mediation function

Supervision is important not only in helping practitioners to be clear about what is expected of them but also as a space to explore their knowledge and understanding about how their role fits with the rest of how services are provided to children. Whether this is their role in the room they are allocated and how children will move from them onto their colleagues in another part of the provision, or their role in preparing children for school, reporting to a child protection case conference or in a looked-after child review (for a child in care). This is the mediation function. Supervision is also the space to explore what the early years practitioner's role is, for example in providing services for a child approaching their two year Integrated Review (the standard review for all children of their health, education, care and development). Depending on the size of the provision, supervisors may have a key role to play in ensuring the demands of owners are understood by practitioners working in different rooms or across a chain of nurseries.

There may also be times when practitioners are seen outside the provision, because they are wearing their uniforms or officially representing the provider, when they have a key role in how the provision is perceived by the local community. Supervisors are required to know how practitioners manage in these settings and how they are behaving when wearing the uniform of the provision. The police investigation that resulted in the serious case review in Plymouth (Nursery Z) began because the practitioner was identified through her uniform.

Checklists which expand on each of these functions are included in the Appendix and provide further clarity about what the differing functions are.

Thinking point

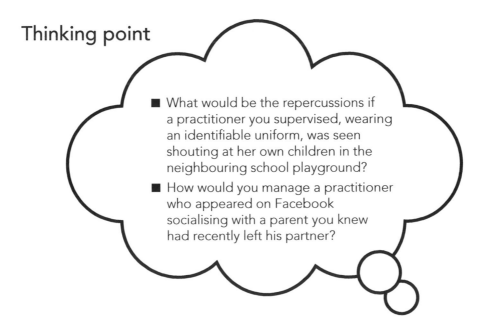

■ What would be the repercussions if a practitioner you supervised, wearing an identifiable uniform, was seen shouting at her own children in the neighbouring school playground?

■ How would you manage a practitioner who appeared on Facebook socialising with a parent you knew had recently left his partner?

Thinking point

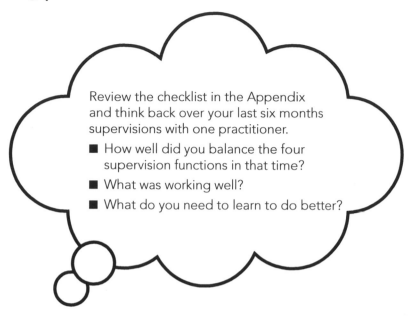

Review the checklist in the Appendix and think back over your last six months supervisions with one practitioner.

■ How well did you balance the four supervision functions in that time?

■ What was working well?

■ What do you need to learn to do better?

The difference between performance appraisal and supervision

Understanding the four functions of supervision helps to clarify what the purpose of supervision is and what it is not. It also makes clear the boundary between supervision and performance appraisal at one end of the spectrum and supervision and counselling at the other (see Figure 1.1). Supervisors need to remain mindful of their need to offer emotional support, not just managerial input (at the performance appraisal end), but equally that their role is to ensure accountability and not only to support and encourage (at the counselling end). Supervisors are not counsellors, nor are they just interested in the performance of practitioners.

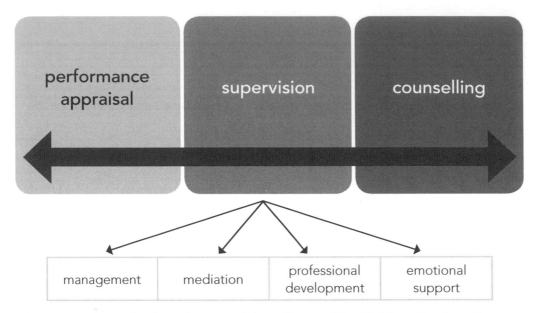

Figure 1.1: Boundaries of supervision. Created by Bridget Rothwell.

One way of thinking about this process as the supervisor is to imagine yourself with stakes set in the ground around supervision and with those stakes your role is to ensure you keep yourself in the middle. Imagine there is a rubber band keeping the stakes together. When you feel yourself being pulled into the performance appraisal box remember the importance of emotional support so that you effectively stretch the imaginary rubber band holding the stakes together but never lean so far over you only assess performance. Nor when pulled in the opposite direction (towards the right of the diagram) do you become the practitioner's counsellor. The idea of the rubber band enforces the flexibility required from the supervisor and, equally, the need for that rubber band to remain intact and unbroken. Practitioners need to know where the stakes in the ground are as well as the supervisor being clear about the remit of their role. There will be times when the rubber band is stretched as practitioners require frequent monitoring around a performance, issue or more intensive support as they deal with a personal crisis. The metaphor of the rubber band is to demonstrate the need for flexibility while remaining able to pull back into shape as quickly as possible and not to pull so hard and often in one direction that it breaks.

An important point here is about the boundary between performance appraisal and supervision. As identified under the management function, there is a clear role for a formal performance appraisal process, at which the practitioner's performance and competence is discussed with them and developmental tasks/goals identified for the future. There will also be occasions when a practitioner's competence or capability raises concern on the part of the supervisor. It is crucial for the trust required by both parties to improve competency, that practitioners understand when their competence is an ongoing part (but never the only focus) of supervision, and when it is being formally appraised. Formal appraisals can run alongside supervision (by being carried out by the same person) but are recommended to be a separate part of the supervisory process. There may be developmental tasks identified as part of a formal appraisal process that supervisors and practitioners discuss in supervision, although the formal evaluation of progress is conducted within the appraisal.

The importance of both performance appraisal and supervision need to be understood. They are both necessary to build awareness of how well a practitioner is working; for the practitioner, their supervisor and the provision in general. Therefore clarity about the boundaries between the two processes has to be maintained by all parties. It is not helpful for performance appraisal to be subsumed within supervision. Performance appraisal is a formal process. Monitoring the tasks identified from a performance appraisal may take place in supervision, however the evaluative process remains separate from it. Sometimes separating the roles of appraiser and supervisor helps if the provision is sufficiently large to have more than one person supervising, although how the findings from both supervision and performance appraisal are integrated (for the purposes of ongoing monitoring) has to be agreed by everyone involved.

Supervisor as coach or mentor

Sometimes the terms mentoring, coaching and supervision are confused. This is especially the case as the guidance for EYFS states that coaching is part of the supervisory process.

> 'Effective supervision provides support, **coaching** and training for the practitioner...'
>
> (Department for Education, 2014, para. 3.19, emphasis added)

The definitions used below highlight what is meant firstly by coaching and secondly by mentoring.

> 'A coach is an individual who helps another identify or remedy performance or skill deficit via modelling and rehearsal.'

> 'A mentor is the person who helps another learn from their experience in the workplace. It is a developmental alliance between equals.'
>
> (Hay, 1995)

It is perfectly legitimate that these activities fit within the supervisor's role. In gaining an understanding of supervision it is essential to accept how the management of a practitioner's work is key to the task of supervision. In supervision the managerial function can never be omitted; a supervisor remains accountable for the standard of work of those they supervise. However, coaching and encouraging practitioners' development are also important functions of supervision. The following image shows how the coaching style supervisors adopt may change as a practitioner develops expertise, from the supervisor being directive with a newer practitioner to allowing a more experienced practitioner scope to move themselves forward in their role while developing their potential.

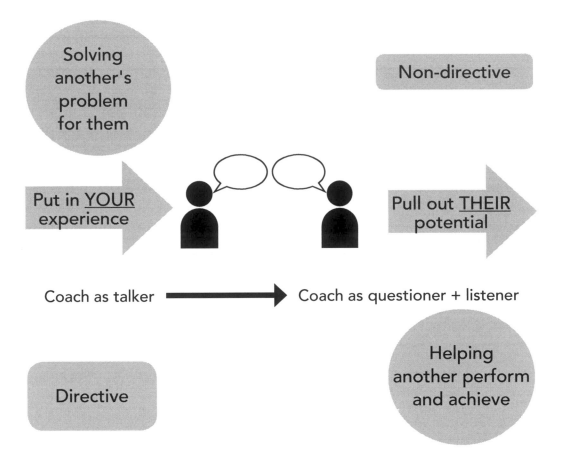

Figure 1.2: Developing coaching skills in supervision. Adapted with permission from Downey M (2003) *Effective Coaching: Lessons from the coach's coach* (2nd edition). London: Cengage Learning.

Sometimes the supervisor may decide that involving others would be of benefit to the practitioner as suggested by the definitions of mentor or coach above. Other elements that support the functions of supervision can be delegated, so a practitioner may be asked to act as mentor to a new staff member joining the provision. For example, a practitioner who needs to be more imaginative in how they encourage children to develop their play could be coached by a more accomplished practitioner. Skilled, effective supervisors will be able to decide whether they are coaching or mentoring the practitioners they are supervising themselves or when they will ask others to act as mentors or coaches for particular elements of the practitioner's job role. This fits well with the EYFS definition about coaching and training being integral to supervision (Department for Education, 2014).

There is further discussion in Chapter 4 about how supervisors recognise and adjust their coaching abilities depending on the competence of the practitioner (supervisee).

Effective supervision has accountability at its core

Supervision has to be very clear where accountability lies, so that when important decisions need to be made, such as whether a child is at immediate risk, it is known who is accountable for decision making. Arguably, it is this clarity around accountability, as opposed to other activities, which defines it as supervision. However the supervisor might well have identified practitioners who are able to build relationships and share their skills, and by pairing them up for specific activities, can facilitate others' professional development. These may be part of the supervisory arrangement or they could be activities delegated by the supervisor to meet the needs of the practitioner. Some nurseries, for example, have room meetings where groups of practitioners work together as peers discussing how to facilitate the children's learning; these meetings may include a supportive element. It is essential that resolution of any difficulties, especially when management clarity is required, and opportunities to reflect on the learning provided in each setting is still part of the ongoing relationship built in supervision (see Chapter 5 for further discussion on this point).

Nursery Z highlighted the often close knit relationship between early years providers, the community they serve, practitioners and parents. When the boundaries and responsibilities are not clear there is scope for children to be harmed. Clarifying boundaries including managerial accountabilities and ensuring practitioners understand their responsibilities and deliver on them is a significant part of supervision.

Because of the nature of the task, the location of providers within small communities and the attraction of working in early years settings for parents who are juggling the demands of caring for children and earning an income, establishing appropriate personal and professional relationships is not always clear cut. Many practitioners working in early years settings began their careers as parent helpers. Others maintain their career once they become parents, by bringing their own children to work with them. The boundaries around each role – practitioners working in the provision, parents leaving children there, parent volunteers or recruited into the workforce – need to be very carefully understood and reinforced, especially where there may be overlaps. Some of the specific challenges facing the early years sector implementing supervision are dealt with in chapter 5. The point here is that all practitioners including volunteers, whether parent helpers or not, require supervision in the spirit of the EYFS guidance.

> *'Providers must put appropriate arrangements in place for the supervision of staff who have contact with children and families.'*
>
> (Department for Education, 2014)

Using the definition of supervision given in this guide it becomes possible to ensure that, regardless of their role, everyone working in the provision understands their task (the management function), how their role could expand (development function), who to talk to about their concerns (support function) and expectations of behaviour within and beyond the provision (mediation function). For practitioners who are also using the provision as parents, this needs to include what will happen should there be concerns about their own child.

How does supervision fit into the EYFS

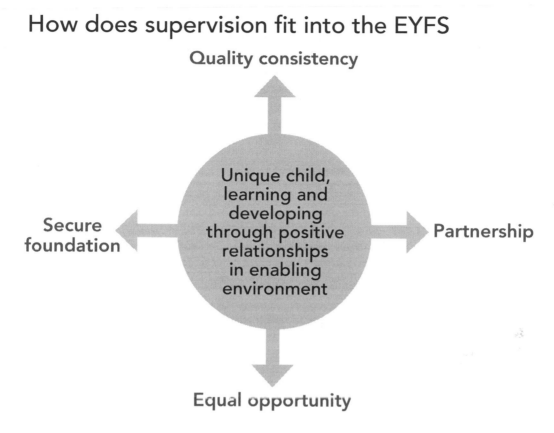

Figure 1.3: Mapping principles of EYFS

Figure 1.3 summarises the overarching principles in the EYFS framework and puts the child at the centre to promote the best outcomes for children using early years settings. The key ideas from the framework are highlighted in the following discussion as the focus of this guide shifts to how supervision happens (Chapter 2). The 4x4x4 model advocated in this manual, which is built on extensive application in social care settings, rests on the importance of a relationship between the supervisor and supervisee. Relationships are at the heart of this model and blend with the ambition of the EYFS framework that promotes positive relationships for children; with their families, the early years provision they attend and the communities in which they are growing up. Understanding what the core components of supervision are and why they are considered core will help early years providers work out what is important to replicate and what they will need to manage differently because of the particular circumstance of their setting. This is discussed in greater detail in Chapter 6. Supervisees have reported greatest satisfaction with supervision when it is based on a trusting relationship with a supervisor (Lambley *et al*, 2013).

For supervision to be taken seriously there has to be agreement within the provision about the importance of supervision and how it will be given priority over other demands (see Chapter 4). As it is a statutory requirement, Ofsted will clearly be looking for evidence that supervision is happening. Supervision records should make clear how the planning around the uniqueness of each child by enabling their learning and development is taking place. Supervision therefore needs to be a formal process that is agreed and negotiated in advance between supervisor and supervisee. However, there will be occasions when other demands intrude and deciding how those will be managed is also an important feature in making supervision effective. As can be seen in the chart below, there are arguments for and against every form of supervision and a flexible response will be required at times based on the supervisor's knowledge of the supervisee, their professional judgement of the situation and the level of risk management required. Formal, planned supervision clearly has greatest benefits for everyone and is recommended as the most frequent form of supervision.

Advantages	Disadvantages
Formal planned supervision ■ Permits advance preparation – agenda, relevant notes/information can be brought, confidential space can be arranged, time allocated. ■ Both people prepared and have already thought about issues leading to better reflection. ■ Review previous decisions and ensure tasks allocated previously have been followed up. ■ Always recorded so clear continuity in the decision making process. ■ Enables monitoring of performance ■ Continuing professional development can be monitored.	■ Less responsive to crisis situations. ■ Some practitioners may prefer more informal meetings. ■ May increase anxiety in less experienced practitioners.
Formal less planned supervision (for example to debrief after a planned action; perhaps attending a review meeting). ■ Planned and responsive to individual need. ■ Reinforces professional learning from planned supervisory session.	■ May need more time than allocated or a confidential space when needed may not be available.

Advantages	Disadvantages
Planned informal session (for example when supervisor responds to request from supervisee for a meeting but sets a time). ■ Allows some preparation for the issue to be discussed. ■ May be appropriately responsive to needs of child and/or supervisee. ■ Nips issues in the bud. ■ There might be a quick solution to an issue that needs resolution.	■ Risks not being fully recorded and the issue might be only partially discussed. ■ Timing and confidentiality likely to be compromised.
Ad-hoc session ('can I just have a quick word?') ■ Suitable response to a crisis when decision needs to be made today. ■ Responsive to emotional needs of supervisee.	■ May not be recorded. ■ Some supervisees will use this as method to avoid supervision. ■ Timing and confidentiality may not allow time for full consideration of issues and lead to poor reactive decision making.

In Chapter 4 there are pro-formas which suggest ideas about what could be included as the basis of supervision agreements which supervisors and supervisees could use to work together. Included within the pro-formas are ideas about how to manage unforeseen events such as absences or crises; it is helpful to talk these issues through at the point of agreeing how to work together.

Thinking point

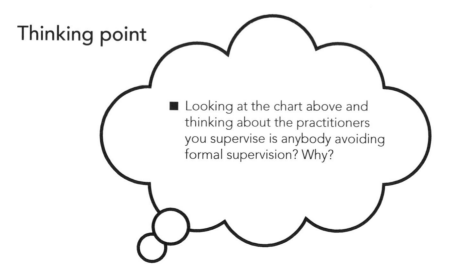

■ Looking at the chart above and thinking about the practitioners you supervise is anybody avoiding formal supervision? Why?

In summary, this chapter has introduced the importance of supervision and why it has become mandatory. It has offered a definition for supervision and explained the main functions of supervision. Terms used in the EYFS guidance have been explained. The importance of supervision and performance appraisal has been emphasised, together with the need for their interdependence. Having addressed the importance of supervision, we move onto considering the core components. The following chapter moves into an explanation of the 4x4x4 model by focusing on the people who are at the heart of the model.

Chapter 2: 4x4x4 model of supervision

Introduction to the 4x4x4 model of supervision

This chapter introduces the 4x4x4 model of supervision. The 4x4x4 model of supervision is the colloquial name for the dominant model of supervisory practice used in social care and has been adapted with input from early years practitioners for use by early years providers. This chapter will explore the meaning of each element and how the core components fit together to provide a model for supervisory practice which is relevant to early years settings.

4x4x4 model of supervision

At the heart of the 4x4x4 model are the key stakeholders in the process. Who benefits from good supervision happening? Child, practitioner, provision and external partners (e.g. parents, health, education). Around the outside of the model are the four functions of supervision discussed in the previous chapter; management, mediation, professional development and emotional support. Core to the model and providing the key links to make this model work is the supervisory cycle. Based on a model of how adults learn, the supervisory cycle assists practitioners to become increasingly skilled and adept at working with children. The detail of how the supervision cycle works is contained in the following chapter with a focus on the links between the layers of the model and their interdependence on each other.

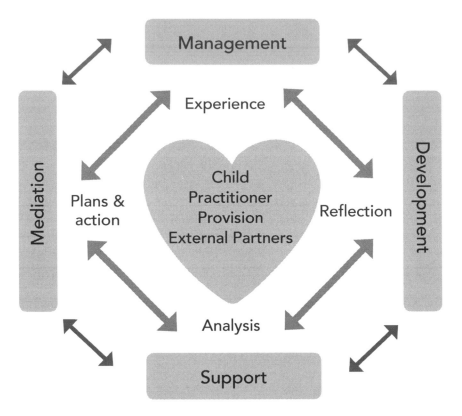

Figure 2.1: 4x4x4 model of supervision. Adapted with permission from Morrison T (2005) *Staff Supervision in Social Care* (3rd edition). Brighton: Pavilion Publishing.

At the heart of the model are the people affected by the quality of supervision; the child or children, practitioners, the provision and interested external parties such as parents, Ofsted, health professionals, school reception teachers and so on. It can be surprising to realise how far the reach of good supervision stretches and, conversely, the reach of poor or no supervision. An interesting activity is to ask practitioners to think about what the likely consequences are of good or poor supervision for each stakeholder in the process. This helps practitioners to understand the significance of supervision and why it matters how effective it is.

Most childcare in early years is provided in group settings by a number of adults. Therefore in considering the child, there will also be knowledge gained from observing the child in the context of their peers and with the opportunity to seek feedback from other practitioners working in the provision with each child. They can be busy, noisy environments at times. In some settings parents may be involved on a daily basis with activities. The stakeholders may have close interdependent relationships and having a space in supervision to reflect may be essential to keeping children safe and observing the signs of children who may need protection.

By using the following hypothetical situation it's possible to unpick how the model can be applied in practice to benefit these key stakeholders.

Case example – Hedgehogs Preschool

Hedgehogs Preschool is situated in a small rural community and has a very good reputation with local parents, and the most recent Ofsted inspection gave it a 'good' grade. The manager of the preschool lives in the village, as do many of the practitioners, and they tend to socialise both within the practitioner group and with parents in the village outside nursery hours. Practitioners are usually recruited by word of mouth and the majority of the team have worked at the preschool for over five years. The administration for the preschool has been undertaken by parent volunteers but lately the main volunteer has left as she has got a permanent job elsewhere. The preschool has recently recruited two new practitioners from outside the area and one of them has been commenting that a lot of attention is paid to one particular child, Maya, by Hannah, one of the supervisors. Hannah is a popular practitioner and the new practitioner has been reassured that this is because Hannah is a friend of Maya's mother. The team have commented that the two new practitioners do not seem to fit in very well and are very rigid in their ideas about childcare practice.

Implications for the child

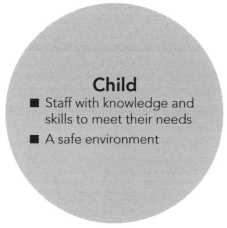

Child
- Staff with knowledge and skills to meet their needs
- A safe environment

There is an indication that Maya, one of the children in the preschool, is receiving particular attention from Hannah, a member of staff. Valuing all children equally and working to include children whatever their needs and abilities is an important feature of the EYFS (Department for Education, 2014, para. 3). Other children could feel excluded from the special attention Hannah gives one of their peers. Maya, who is receiving additional attention, may not be being exposed to the range of opportunities available throughout the setting or helped to make transitions to less familiar adults. Listening to the observations from the new practitioners gives the supervisor an opportunity to review the contact between Hannah and Maya to see how well it fits with the overarching principles of EYFS about assisting children in forming positive relationships, as well as whether the provision is meeting its commitment to equality of opportunity for all children (Department for Education, 2014, para. 6).

Additionally, consideration must be given to the risks of an inappropriate or grooming relationship developing. The serious case reviews into nurseries have highlighted how workers were able to nurture special relationships with children, which led to opportunities to abuse the trust the child had placed in them. Other practitioners, while experiencing disquiet about what they observed to be happening, did not know how to raise their concern (Plymouth Safeguarding Children Board, 2010). In this example the close relationship the new practitioners have observed between Maya and Hannah has been explained as Hannah being a friend of Maya's mother, rather than exploring whether it is a positive relationship for Maya.

Supervision is an opportunity to review each child's progress in their learning journey and to see whether they are being encouraged to take part in the full range of the curriculum. This is also another way in which Maya's needs can be reviewed; does she seek Hannah out as an alternative to trying out new activities or going to less familiar adults?

Therefore the benefits to the child of good supervision are that the provision becomes a safe, enabling environment in which she can learn and develop. Additionally, practitioners have skills to assist in her learning and development as well as safeguard her from harm.

Thinking point

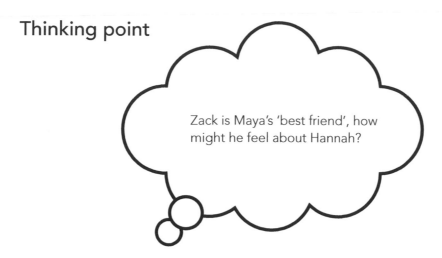

Zack is Maya's 'best friend', how might he feel about Hannah?

Implications for the practitioner

Practitioner

- Clarification of job role and expectations
- A place to discuss concerns and anxieties
- Identification of learning and development needs

The obvious issue arising in this example is managing the boundary between personal and professional relationships. This is a challenging area in the early years environment. Many practitioners started their professional roles in early years settings as parent helpers and evolved into professionals. Community based settings might want to actively recruit practitioners from among the local community. Therefore, understanding the practitioner role and its responsibilities is a significant area of practitioner development. It is daunting for practitioners to manage the boundary between being friends with parents who use the provision and being the professional practitioner in the context of work. It is important that Hannah explores how her friendships outside the provision are managed within, explicitly with Maya and her mother:

- How does she ensure she treats children fairly?

- What information does she pass back to Maya's mother about what is happening in the provision?

- How does she use her relationship with Maya to further Maya's development without negatively impacting on how she may be perceived by other children and their parents?

Supervision is an important place to explore Hannah's values around how she behaves with children she knows from the community, especially in relation to safeguarding them, as she needs to remain vigilant to signs of children being at risk of abuse and neglect (Department for Education, 2014, para. 3.4).
For the two newer practitioners there are issues for them about how to raise concerns and see them properly considered:

- How do they find out about the whistleblowing policy and who they should contact if they have concerns about another practitioner?

- How do the issues they raise around professional boundaries get discussed?

- How do they challenge effectively rather than being ignored as outsiders?

They will also require supervision to explore how they translate their professional knowledge into practice.

Therefore, the implications for practitioners are that supervision is a place to clarify the expectations of the role and what responsibilities are reasonable. Supervision becomes a space to reflect on observations and make sense of experiences, an opportunity to raise concerns. It is also a space in which learning and development needs can be identified and a plan worked out for how they will be met.

Thinking point

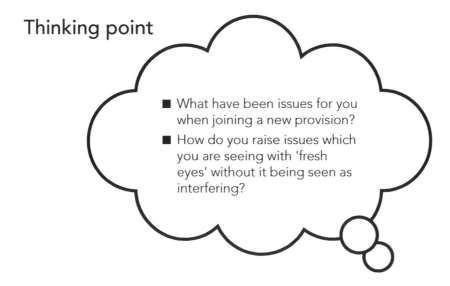

- What have been issues for you when joining a new provision?
- How do you raise issues which you are seeing with 'fresh eyes' without it being seen as interfering?

Implications for the provision

Provision

- Facilities internal communication
- Disseminates agency goals and values
- Contributes to a safe team culture
- Provides information about staff knowledge and skills
- Lowers rates of sickness and turnover

It is obvious that Hedgehogs Preschool in the case study example is not following the EYFS guidance about the safer recruitment of staff and the ongoing responsibility for ensuring that practitioners are suitable as *'practitioners tend to be recruited by word of mouth'*. Understandably there could be consequences for the provision of this and therefore supervision becomes a method of protecting the provision and ensuring its vision and standards are being consistently implemented.

The policies and procedures in relation to safeguarding, child protection, recruitment and induction do not appear to be being implemented. The 'good' assessment by Ofsted may indicate that the policies are in place, yet questions remain about how well they are understood and implemented by practitioners. The boundary around parent volunteers and early years practitioners is not delineated and there are reports that administration is done by parent volunteers and that the workers and parents socialise together.

Finding ways of developing positive relationships with parents is necessary for the ongoing success of early years providers, therefore cultivating and seeking feedback from parents about whether the provision is delivering good quality care to their children is essential. Bring known by parents for delivering this is a key factor in getting repeat business. If parents begin to mistrust the safety of the boundaries between practitioners and parents and have issues about how confidential information is treated, this will affect the reputation of the setting and potentially future viability.

The governance of preschools is another area where greater clarity is required. However, in terms of recommending good supervisory practice, each provider needs to be clear (written into policies which are agreed by committee and practitioners) what needs to be known by committee members and what needs to remain confidential within the provision. In this example there has been a reliance on parent volunteers to assist with the administration and their role with regard to keeping children's information confidential is unclear. The boundaries between the provision and parents are also unclear as there is reported to be social contact. Is there a shared understanding about the boundaries around confidentiality, whistle blowing, making complaints and what the consequences could be? Nursery Z highlights the vulnerability of children in provisions where the personal/professional boundaries have become muddled and where professional responsibility is not clearly understood, especially in relation to child protection (Plymouth Safeguarding Children's Board, 2010).

The role of supervision is an important one to the provision. It gives information about how well the culture of the provision is being understood, especially about how policies and procedures are being followed. Practitioners have an opportunity to reflect on their role in the provision and identify gaps in their skills which providers need to find ways of meeting. The opportunity to offload their emotional concerns lowers rates of sickness and assists in keeping staff motivated. Supervision can be likened to an early warning system; practitioners are encouraged to raise practice issues when they notice them and in discussion in supervision identify more effective ways of working.

Thinking point

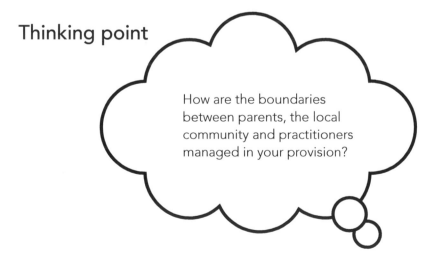

How are the boundaries between parents, the local community and practitioners managed in your provision?

Implications for external partners

External partners
- Increased confidence in quality of care
- Improved communication and relationships

Providers need to have methods of evaluating children's progress and occasions to ensure there is equality of opportunity. Questions that could be asked around the issues arising from the case example are along the following lines:

- What happens to the children of parents who do not socialise or participate on the committee?

- Where are the boundaries of confidentiality; are some parents included inappropriately in knowing information about other children?

- Would parents who are unable/unwilling to join in the social activities feel that their child is at an unequal disadvantage and how could the provision reassure them?

This example raises questions about how well the anti-discriminatory policy is understood and disseminated. The importance of building safe cultures so that the opportunities do not arise for speculative abuse of children have been highlighted in the serious case reviews, and these considerations should be thought about in this context too. If members of the community had concerns about children or practitioners' behaviour how would the manager make sure they could be contacted to listen to their worries? By following procedures and policies and having them available for practitioners, parents and other agencies, the boundaries around behavioural expectations become much clearer.

In summary, supervision helps the communication with external partners about the provision and the quality of care available to children.

Thinking point

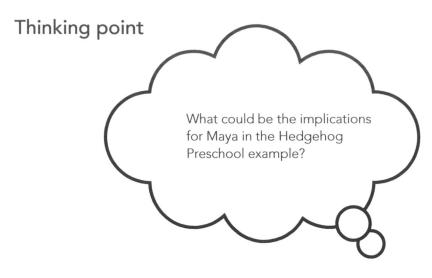

What could be the implications for Maya in the Hedgehog Preschool example?

Child
- Staff with knowledge and skills to meet their needs
- A safe environment

Provision
- Facilitates internal communication
- Disseminates agency goals and values
- Contributes to a safe team culture
- Provides information about staff knowledge and skills
- Lowers rates of sickness and turnover

Why is supervision in early years important?

Practitioner
- Clarification of job role and expectations
- A place to discuss concerns and anxieties
- Identification of learning and development needs

External partners
- Increased confidence in quality of care
- Improved communication and relationships

Figure 2.2: Impact of supervision in early years

Without supervision these opportunities to build quality into the provision may get overlooked. Including difference and managing diversity is an important way of improving quality. The challenge in the example used would be to retain and value the perspective of the newer practitioners and to take an opportunity to review practice through the lens of equal opportunity. It is also a chance to develop practitioners who may have become accustomed to their way of doing things and are resistant to changing to develop their skills and professional interests to better meet children's learning needs.

So at the heart of the 4x4x4 model in Figure 2.1 are the children and the people who care about them. Good supervision reinforces the importance of the quality of relationships practitioners build with the children and their families, their peers and their colleagues outside the setting. This is one of the overarching principles of EYFS (Department for Education, 2014, para. 6).

Still thinking about the dilemmas posed from the Hedgehogs Preschool, our focus shifts to the supervisory functions to demonstrate how the heart of the model links to the outer rim (see Figure 2.1).

The management function

Exploring Hannah's relationship with Maya allows discussion about personal and professional relationships. There may be benefits for Maya of knowing one of the practitioners; this prior knowledge can help her to manage the transition to a new environment, however Hannah needs to think about the quality of her relationship with all the children, not only Maya. Hannah can use supervision to make sense of her role.

- How does she understand the differences between Hannah at nursery and Hannah at home?

- What does Maya's mother expect of Hannah?

- What are the possible conflicts of interest between her role as an early years practitioner and as a family friend?

The supervisor needs to know that practitioners are able to fulfil the expectations of EYFS. Supervision can be a space to decide whether Hannah should have the key work role with Maya or that be allocated to another practitioner.

- How will Hannah manage either role?

- How able would she feel in reporting child protection concerns about a friend?

Similarly the management function of supervision is important in using the insight and feedback gained from fresh perspectives when new practitioners join, and their induction process will be an opportunity to explore their knowledge, skills and value base to ensure that high quality, consistent care to children is maintained. How can their experience and knowledge gained from working in other places add to the team's skills? Supervision provides a vehicle for assessing the competence of new practitioners and the structure of making induction tasks manageable.

The mediation function

Some of the issues previously discussed might well come into this function as part of supervision is to explore with the practitioner the consequences of their behaviour inside and outside the provision. For instance, if Hannah is known by other parents to be a particularly good friend of Maya's mother, how will this affect their use of the nursery and their ability to trust Hannah? The provision needs to be very clear about the policies around the boundary between social friendships and professional accountability. Social media policies and professional codes of conduct should be essential to the setting, however it becomes part of supervision to ensure their meaning is understood and adhered to. The advantage of having this function as key to supervision is that it enables the practitioner to think about how this behaviour might be perceived by someone else, for example an Ofsted inspector.

Professional development function

In the Hedgehogs example there is a difference of view being expressed about childcare practice. Exploring the nature of such differences and helping practitioners to keep up to date with how childcare practices change is an important task of supervision. Identifying learning and developmental goals and finding opportunities to build those into the role is also important. Professional development incorporates informal opportunities as well as formal learning opportunities. Supervisors may know which practitioner is imaginative in involving children in exploring their environment and which practitioner prefers to avoid messier activities. Building learning alliances between peers as discussed in the previous chapter can be part of the coaching or mentoring tasks supervisors allocate to supervisees. The new practitioners at Hedgehogs potentially provide developmental opportunities for more experienced practitioners to learn about recent research while experienced practitioners will have a good working knowledge of the children and may, for example, use effective techniques in getting reluctant children to try new activities.

Emotional support function

It may be anticipated that this situation for the new staff has emotional content. Joining a group, especially one that is established, raises issues about being inside or outside the group. When the situation like the one described here suggests a dominant culture of inclusivity it is not easy for outsiders to join in; newcomers may find the culture 'cliquey' and can feel judged and disliked. Should the situation include elements of diversity it is critical that supervision becomes a space in which to explore difference. However there is no mention of the cultural component in the description. Should one of the new practitioners be white British and attempting to join a black British practitioner team, for example, it should be explored whether the resistance to their new ideas has any basis in their difference from the rest of the team. Similarly a male practitioner joining a female staff team may have different needs which he should be able to explore in supervision. Sheryl Sandberg, chief operating officer of Facebook described in a TED talk how in a meeting she asked to use the toilet only to discover that no one in the meeting (she was the only woman present) knew where the ladies toilets were, because they had never needed to know. What would an all-female team assume about the needs of a man?

Learning to ask practitioners about the emotional impact the work has on them is a skill supervisors need to learn as well as how to establish the trust that makes it possible to explore emotionally charged issues. Being cared about is a strong reason why people continue to work where they do.

Thinking point

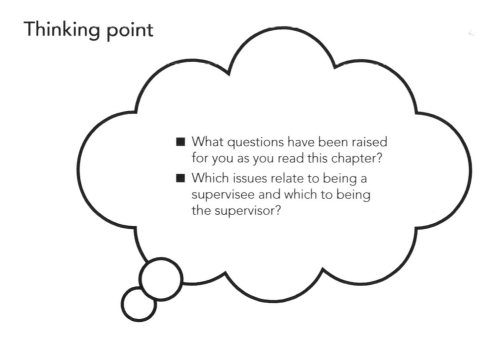

- What questions have been raised for you as you read this chapter?
- Which issues relate to being a supervisee and which to being the supervisor?

This chapter has introduced the 4x4x4 model for supervisory practice by introducing the key stakeholders – the people at the heart of the model who benefit from effective supervision. The model incorporates the functions of supervision introduced in the previous chapter and also shows how the link between the two layers is provided by the supervisory cycle. The supervisory cycle is the subject of the next chapter.

Chapter 3: The supervision cycle

Introduction

The supervision cycle holds the 4x4x4 model together. It binds the heart of the model (the people who benefit) to the outer rim (the functions supervision performs) by finding a way of allowing practitioners space and time in which to reflect on and learn from their working experience. This chapter is going to focus on the importance of understanding the theory that underpins the supervision cycle. By using a case example it will show how the theory can be applied to practice. This will also make clear how the model fits with the expectations of EYFS (Department for Education, 2014) about supervision.

The supervision cycle

The supervision cycle is a model adapted by Tony Morrison (2005) and others (Davys & Beddoe, 2012; Wonnacott, 2012; 2014) from Kolb's learning cycle (Kolb, 1988). Kolb's work about how adults learn draws on the essential components of observing, feeling, thinking and doing. In learning new skills there needs to be an understanding of the theory of the skill, to learn why what you are trying to do may work and why it may not, often by being shown. In learning any new skill there are emotional components; how you feel in trying something new (especially if you consider you might fail at it), and the opportunity to both try it out and think about how it could be improved. Importantly, these processes need to be repeated and reviewed. In order to understand the process of supervision it can be helpful to reflect on how adults learn.

Jane wants to learn to crochet. She is good at knitting and enjoys craft activities. However, one thing Jane knows is that often when she goes to an adult education class the teacher is right handed and she is left handed, so it can be harder to master skills. Sandra suggests learning from YouTube and Jane discovers Sandra is correct; there are tuition tutorials which are for left handers. Jane watches them through for a bit and notices there is one which is filmed so that the camera angle is as if looking down at the work so she can copy the hand placement. Jane decides to follow this tutorial and buys the necessary equipment. The tutorial is very good, Jane can stop it when she needs to check out the hand placement and she can see that what she is doing matches what is being shown. Jane feels very proud at completing the piece of work shown on the video.

Contrast this example with the one below.

Mike has been challenged by his mates to try unicycling. He's fit and athletic and knows he has good balance on a bike. In the context of his group of friends Mike is the qualified sports instructor and the expectation from them and himself is that it will be easy for him to unicycle because he has transferable skills. Mike falls off repeatedly to the amusement of his friends and walks away demoralised vowing never to try again.

What similarities and differences are there in the two examples and how may they be relevant to the supervision cycle? In both examples Jane and Mike have past experience which is relevant but not identical to the new skill they want to learn. Mike has done what is often referred to as a 'quick fix'; he's assumed that because he has all the knowledge he needs from riding a normal bike, as he has good balance and is athletic, that he can do unicycling without understanding how it works and differs from a normal bike. Yes, he had relevant past experience, but he went straight to doing without any thinking about what he needed to do differently and how he might feel.

In a quiet moment perhaps Mike could be persuaded to try it out again if he asked for help from his peers or a trainer in getting his balance on the unicycle and had a better understanding of the theory of unicycling. Mike needed emotional support and a better grasp of the theory to succeed in riding a unicycle – the elements of the learning cycle he skipped over.

Jane used her past experiences to recognise that she needed different tuition. To learn crocheting it was essential that she found someone to guide her who was also left handed. With the support of a friend she found a video tutorial, and after watching it through Jane decided that she had sufficient understanding of the process to risk buying some wool and hooks to try it out for herself. Jane felt sufficiently confident and supported to try a new experience. She watched another person demonstrate, using their left hand as she needed to do herself, so she understood the theory of how to use the hook and the wool to make a crochet mat. Jane tried it out and succeeded.

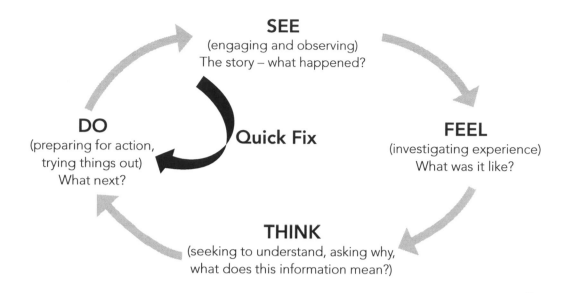

Figure 3.1: 'Quick fix' cycle – missing out feeling and thinking. Reprinted with permission from Morrison T (2005) *Staff Supervision in Social Care.* Brighton: Pavilion Publishing & Media

The significance of these examples is the importance of every element of the learning cycle in effective learning. It is possible for people to copy others and replicate what they have seen. However, if they do not understand why they are doing what they are, they may run into difficulty if they encounter a different situation; for example people who have learnt to ski without understanding how to stop.

Learning new skills takes time and practice. All elements need to happen for skills to be learnt, however, they will not necessarily happen in the same order for everyone. As Kolb developed his theory he identified that people appear to have a preference for a learning style and therefore to start learning in different places on the cycle.

Thinking point

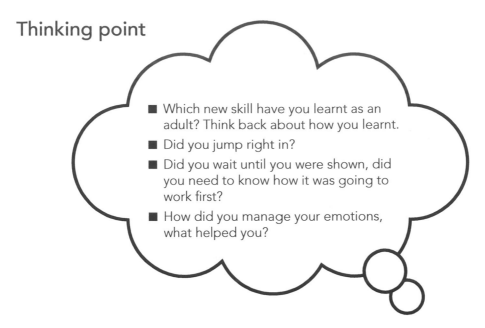

- Which new skill have you learnt as an adult? Think back about how you learnt.
- Did you jump right in?
- Did you wait until you were shown, did you need to know how it was going to work first?
- How did you manage your emotions, what helped you?

Mike from the previous example is an activist (seeing); he likes to learn by trying things out. However he needs to be helped to recognise that managing his emotions when he does not succeed and learning to find out why, are also required for effective learning. Jane likes to understand the theory before she starts to learn a new skill; she starts the learning cycle as a theorist (thinker). For her the challenge at times will be about taking a risk and trying something before she has completely grasped the theory.

In both the above examples, the quality of the support affected whether the adult learnt their new skill. Kolb's learning theory (1988) is therefore a good fit with supervision. The aim of supervision is that practitioners understand what is expected as part of their job role, are able to deliver acceptable standards of practice, that they question why things happen, know when and how to act on what they see within or outside the provision and are able to reflect on and learn from their experiences with the support of their supervisor. Thus the supervision cycle matches the functions of supervision; management, mediation, professional development and emotional support.

Experience SEE
(engaging and observing)
The story – what happened?

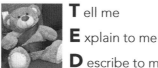

T ell me
E xplain to me
D escribe to me

Action Plans DO
(preparing for action,
trying things out)
What next?

Reflection FEEL
(investigating experience)
What was it like?

Analysis THINK
(seeking to understand, asking why,
what does this information mean?)

Figure 3.2: The supervision cycle. Adapted with permission from Morrison T (2005) Staff Supervision in Social Care. Brighton: Pavilion

Supervision promotes the activities in early years environments which encourage children to move forward in their learning and development. Supervision is a method of encouraging professional development. It therefore mirrors a major task of the early years environments, to facilitate children's development. Practitioners may observe children going through phases of the learning cycle themselves trying to work out why things are happening, for example building a tower of bricks. Practitioners are expected to question whether the child is making the progress they would anticipate, and if not why not, so that the reasons can be addressed and the child assisted in moving on.

Figure 3.2 shows the supervision cycle with the processes described as seeing, feeling, thinking and doing. Supervision is a collaborative relationship between supervisor and supervisee with the aim of empowering the supervisee to develop as a practitioner. Using the supervision cycle takes a supervisee through a reflective process in which the supervisor encourages them to think about their work, or a specific child. Each process is explored a little bit further to clarify how supervision works.

Experience/'seeing'

The experience part of the cycle helps the practitioner and supervisor to gather information about the child; their family situation, the observations the practitioner has made, comments they have heard from others and so on. Its purpose is an information gathering process. From the supervisor's open questions, practitioners are encouraged to think about all the sources of information they have about that child and their current situation. It is important that consideration is given to the perspectives of others.

Reflection/'feeling'

Within the reflective part of the cycle is the opportunity to explore emotions. Children, especially when pre-verbal or traumatised, may well show emotions that have a powerful impact on other people without always being able to identify what is causing their distress. Practitioners will have their own childhood histories and occasionally those experiences may impact on a current situation. They need to be aware of how their reactions from their own situation are affecting their ability to think about this child's situation now.

Practitioners will also be experiencing life stressors to varying degrees and need to be helped to remain alert to the impact of these issues on their performance, including their responsivity to the children. This element of the supervision cycle is a space for the practitioner to reflect on their emotional responses to their work. The supervisor asks questions that prompt the practitioner to delve into their emotional reactions to their key children and how they are experiencing working in the provision.

Probing in this way may raise issues around practitioner's views and beliefs which affect how they feel about undertaking all the responsibilities of their role. It is also an opportunity to ask the practitioner how the child is feeling and whether they have noticed changes in how others are caring for or about the child, which the child may be responding to.

Analysis/'thinking'

The analysis part of the cycle is seeking to make sense of the information and drawing on knowledge and theories that the supervisor and supervisee may have. There may be a range of possible explanations emerging and all may need consideration rather than only thinking about one. In fact, encouraging practitioners to explore a range of possibilities to explain what they have seen is important to meet the aims of EYFS of confirming children are developing in their own unique way. It is also essential that children's safety is reviewed. Supervisors can use this part of the cycle to ensure practitioners have up-to-date knowledge about child development and know what they are looking for in assessing children's learning and safety. Supervisors at this part of the cycle may find it helpful to use the perspective of another party to allow different theories or viewpoints to emerge. Practitioners need to join in this part to explain what they think is happening and in preparation for thinking about what they should do next.

Action planning/'doing'

When reaching this part of the cycle there is a great temptation for the supervisor to come up with a list of actions, however the key to successful professional development is enabling the practitioner to work out their own action plan from the questions the supervisor asks. There are several reasons for urging supervisors to resist from fixing the problems their supervisees bring. Firstly, practitioners need to develop their own problem solving abilities. Secondly, when practitioners come up with their own solutions, they are more likely to take the responsibility for implementing them. Thirdly, and significantly, supervisors gain information about the competence of the practitioner. Developing practitioners' abilities to think through the consequences of situations in this way enables them to become more professionally autonomous and prepares them for taking on additional responsibilities. It also lessens the demands made on supervisors to sort problems out.

Thinking point

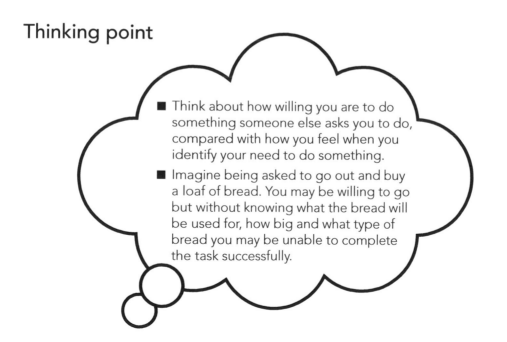

- Think about how willing you are to do something someone else asks you to do, compared with how you feel when you identify your need to do something.
- Imagine being asked to go out and buy a loaf of bread. You may be willing to go but without knowing what the bread will be used for, how big and what type of bread you may be unable to complete the task successfully.

The art for the supervisor is to facilitate an environment in which the supervisee will best be able to learn. Recognising the emotional state of the supervisee is important in the first instance and attention needs to be given to attuning to the supervisee's emotional state and building rapport sufficiently that safety in the supervisory process is established. So supposing supervision begins where both participants are feeling prepared and calm, how does the supervisor facilitate a learning environment for the supervisee? The ted(dy) bear picture in Figure 3.2 is a clue. The T.E.D. questions that are used to facilitate children's development are transferable to adult learning environments; Tell me, Explain to me, Describe to me.

The art of good, effective supervision is asking open questions

This sounds simple, until supervisors try out resisting their urge to fix problems. Often when new to management roles there is a belief that being a manager requires coming up with the answers. This is hard to resist especially if practitioners bring this expectation with them, with statements such as '*As my manager, I expect you to tell me what to do*'. Supervisors, remembering that the functions and reach of supervision goes beyond themselves and their supervisee, can usefully spend time practising their skills in asking open questions.

Using the supervision cycle in practice

The following example allows supervisors to understand how the supervision cycle works in practice. It also demonstrates how the cycle fits within the 4x4x4 model.

Case example – Cottontails Nursery

Cottontails Nursery is situated in a suburb of a large town and serves a wide geographical area with pockets of deprivation and high unemployment. Several of the children in the nursery are funded by the local authority. There is a large staff group of very committed early years practitioners who are highly skilled at helping the children to achieve their full potential. They know that many of the parents they are working with have not had an easy life and struggle to make ends meet. Tanya is two years old and regularly comes to the nursery saying she is hungry. Practitioners will always give her something to eat as they know her mother often leaves the house early in the morning to get to her cleaning job, and Tanya's aunt, age 16, looks after her in the morning and brings her to nursery. Tanya's mother always picks Tanya up and there is obviously real affection between the two. Recently, on one or two occasions, Joanne, one of the practitioners has thought she smelt alcohol on Mum's breath.

Joanne comes to supervision saying she would like to talk about Tanya but it is 'probably nothing'.

As Joanne's supervisor how would you explore this with her?

Suggested questions to ask about <u>experience</u> might include the following:
- Tell me what 'probably nothing' is?

- Tell me more about your concerns for Tanya?

- What else have you seen?

- Who else is concerned about Tanya?

- What have you noticed?

- When did you start to notice these things?

- How has Mum appeared to you?

- Describe Tanya's relationship with her aunt.

- How is Tanya managing here in the nursery?

Suggested questions to ask about <u>reflection</u> might include the following:
- How do you feel?

- How do you think Tanya feels?

- How do you feel about Mum?

- How do you feel about Tanya?

- How do other practitioners feel about Tanya?

- Have you encountered similar situations in the past, how did you feel then?

- What is making you feel anxious?

- Who else is worried about Tanya?

- What upsets you most about Tanya's situation?

Suggested questions to ask about <u>analysis</u> might include the following:
- What do you think Tanya needs at the moment?

- How would you assess Tanya developmentally?

- What is working well in this family?

- What support do you think this family needs?

- Who is at risk in this family?

- What risks are there?

- What explanations do you have for what you have observed?

- How do you think Mum is managing?

- How do you know Tanya is safe at home?

Suggested questions to ask about <u>action planning</u> might include the following:
- What do you think needs to happen next?

- What will meet Tanya's needs?

- Who needs to do it?

- What support do you need?

- How will you decide whether to involve other agencies?

- When should we review this plan?

- What would make you more or less concerned about Tanya?

Applying the 4x4x4 model to practice

If the supervision cycle was adhered to as above the supervisor would have asked Joanne to discuss her emotional responses to Tanya and helped her to evaluate, by using her knowledge and observations, whether her concern was 'probably nothing' or had some evidence to it. She would have been allowed to test out her hypotheses about what might be happening to Tanya and asked to consider the viewpoints of Tanya, her mother, her aunt and other practitioners before forming a plan about what to do next.

The functions of supervision would have been met in the following ways. The supervisor would finish with a clear action plan including timescales and desirable outcomes that were recorded on the child's file. The supervisee would know what is expected of her and by when. Therefore the management function of supervision would be met. Joanne would have been asked to think about the role of the nursery and when to involve other agencies. She would be asked to form a view about whether there is evidence of Tanya being at risk of abuse or neglect and to think about her child protection responsibilities to Tanya. These form part of the mediation role. Joanne would have been offered the space to think over her previous experiences and what developmental needs she might have for further learning or coaching in acquiring new skills. This is the developmental function. There has been space to review the emotional impact on Joanne of her concerns about Tanya and for her to consider what specific support needs she has. This is the support function of supervision.

The heart of the model is about the people who are affected by supervision. In this example Joanne's role as the practitioner in working with Tanya, the child, was explored. Consideration also expanded to the relationship the nursery (provision) had with Tanya, other members of her family and Joanne, as well as its responsibilities to work with other partner agencies in safeguarding and promoting Tanya's well-being.

> *'3.21: Providers must put appropriate arrangements in place for the supervision of staff who have contact with children and families. Effective supervision provides support, coaching and training for the practitioner and promotes the interests of children...*
>
> *3.22: Supervision should provide opportunities for staff to:*
> - *Discuss any issues – particularly concerning children's development or well-being;*
> - *Identify solutions to address issues as they arise; and*
> - *Receive coaching to improve their personal effectiveness.'*

(Expectations of supervision from EYFS, Department for Education, 2014)

Again using the example of Joanne's supervision process, she has been offered an opportunity to discuss Tanya, her development and her emotional well-being including whether there are any child protection concerns. Through the discussion, questions were asked about Joanne's development needs and the opportunity to identify training needs. Joanne was also expected to look for and identify solutions to the issue she brought about her concern for Tanya.

The role of emotions within supervision

Implicit within the supervisory relationship is an awareness and respect for practitioners' emotional needs. Goleman (1995) described the importance of emotional intelligence for the social life human beings share together. Relationships shape our development. Early years practitioners are already familiar with how relationships shape a child's world and are encouraged to use positive relationships with the child to stimulate their development (Department for Education, 2014; Gerhardt, 2004; Sunderland, 2007).

An understanding of these concepts is helpful and transfers across into supervision. Morrison (2007) described this as the emotional intelligence paradigm. The supervisor is aware of their own emotional responses and is able to manage them (intrapersonal relationship). Therefore the supervisor consciously thinks before supervision about their own emotional state and notices how they are feeling. If they become aware that there are feelings aroused by working with a supervisee, the supervisor prepares for this by thinking about why and how they plan to address it. The supervisor takes responsibility for being self-aware and arriving for supervision emotionally regulated. Within the relationship with a supervisee the emotionally intelligent supervisor is alert to how the other person (the supervisee) is feeling and able to use this awareness, sometimes called empathy, in managing the relationship between them (interpersonal relationship). This is portrayed in Figure 3.3 below.

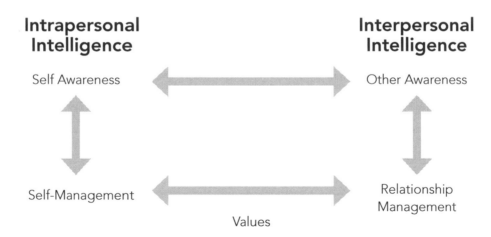

Figure 3.3: The emotional intelligence paradigm

Importantly, underpinning the foundations of ethical supervisory practice is an explicit agreement between the participants about the values they share. The EYFS framework has clear values that form part of the over-arching principles and these may be referenced in the agreement between each party in the supervision process (Department for Education, 2014).

Recognising the impact of anxiety within supervision

While supervisors will be alert to the range of emotional responses supervisees display it is worth acknowledging the impact that anxiety may have, as it can be particularly destabilising in the context of a work environment. Anxiety may stimulate the brain into 'doing mode' (fight or flight responses). When children get hyper aroused practitioners will be good at soothing and settling them by gradually explaining what they are doing or what will be happening, for example *'Mummy will be coming after snack time'*. Supervisors will be developing their emotional radar by picking up clues about how practitioners and children are responding to situations and using those as cues to guide supervision. It can be tempting sometimes, especially if feeling rushed or under pressure to make a decision, for a supervisor to go straight from seeing to doing and skipping the feeling and thinking stages. This may be likened to a 'quick fix'. In a similar way when Mike tried the 'quick fix' method of learning to unicycle, it resulted in a less successful outcome than if he had asked for the support he needed to learn and the theory of how to balance and ride the unicycle. As supervisors, the skill is to build on this awareness so that you facilitate a practitioner's ability to manage her emotional reactions. Supervisors want practitioners to think about the consequences of what they have seen that provoked anxiety in them and what other explanations there could be, besides the one that has made them anxious.

Sometimes this pressure to make decisions quickly to shift the anxiety, for example about a child's safety, is hard for supervisors to resist. A very experienced supervisor once explained that she always had 'a cup of tea moment' when she was being pressured by practitioners into hasty decision making. Taking a breathing space allows the body and emotions a space to calm which allows the thinking processes to be activated. The experience of making a drink helps the supervisor to prepare emotionally for what they could be dealing with, it gives a supervisee an opportunity to spend a few minutes reviewing what they want to say and, because they feel cared about, increases their ability to self-regulate.

This is summarised in Figure 3.4. The three layers are a simplistic design of the doing, feeling and thinking layers of the brain. The doing layer is the brainstem where the rush to action is located, often referred to as fight or flight. The ability to understand and respond to feelings is located within the limbic layer and the thinking layer is the cortex.

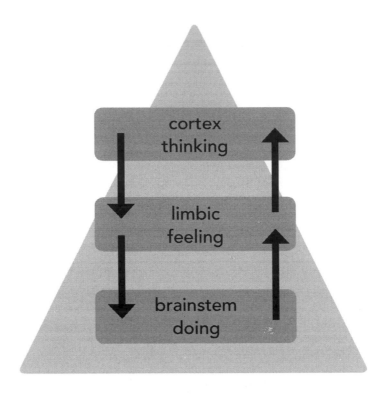

Figure 3.4: Helping practitioners self-regulate

So the 'cup of tea moment' consciously allows the supervisor and supervisee to move away from reacting/doing, the act of caring for each other settles the feeling layer and as the anxiety lessens and the care for each other gets activated it also allows the thinking part of the brain to take over. Sometimes referred to as 'bottom up/top down' management of an anxiety-inducing state, supervisors need to recognise these processes consciously and consider how to manage practitioners who have moved into a fight or flight mode of behaving. Early years practitioners have great experience at facilitating this process with toddlers who are beginning to experience strong feelings and need to be helped by being given language and explanations that soothe their anxiety. It is essential that supervisors don't get drawn into fight or flight tactics when presented with this by supervisees and address the feeling and thinking layers before taking action.

Thinking point

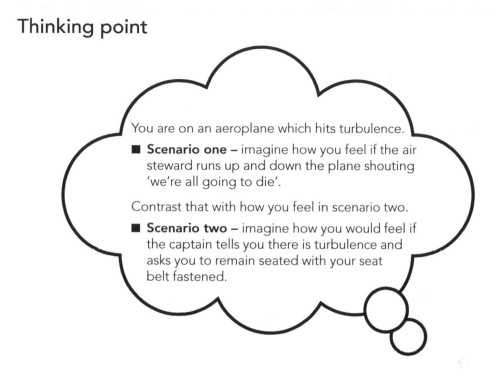

You are on an aeroplane which hits turbulence.

- **Scenario one** – imagine how you feel if the air steward runs up and down the plane shouting 'we're all going to die'.

Contrast that with how you feel in scenario two.

- **Scenario two** – imagine how you would feel if the captain tells you there is turbulence and asks you to remain seated with your seat belt fastened.

Supervisors are effectively the captains of the aeroplane and supervision becomes the method for managing the emotional and thinking responses of the practitioners within the provision.

Within this chapter the 4x4x4 model of supervision has been shown working in practice. The 4x4x4 model fits the expectations of EYFS for supervision. The 4x4x4 model of supervision benefits the people at its heart. However, the essence of this chapter was to explore how adults learn, and using the learning cycle as its base, how the supervision cycle maps onto adults' experiences of learning and development. Some of the pitfalls of skipping stages of the learning cycle have been pointed out and the dangers of managers becoming too directive highlighted. The key messages to take away are the art of open questioning and the importance of being emotionally attuned as a supervisor. The next chapter focuses on negotiating and fulfilling the role of an authoritative, effective supervisor.

Chapter 4: Authoritative supervision – agreeing and recording reflective supervision

Introduction

In this chapter the concept of the authoritative supervisor is introduced as well as ideas about power and authority that underpin effective authoritative supervisory practice; specifically, the importance of agreeing the terms under which supervision is conducted, the significance of a supervision agreement and the process by which the agreement and subsequent supervisions are recorded. Also included within the chapter are templates to assist these processes.

The authoritative supervisor

The authoritative supervisor understands their role, is comfortable with using authority when they need to, and has high expectations of practitioners, while remaining emotionally attuned to the needs of their supervisee.

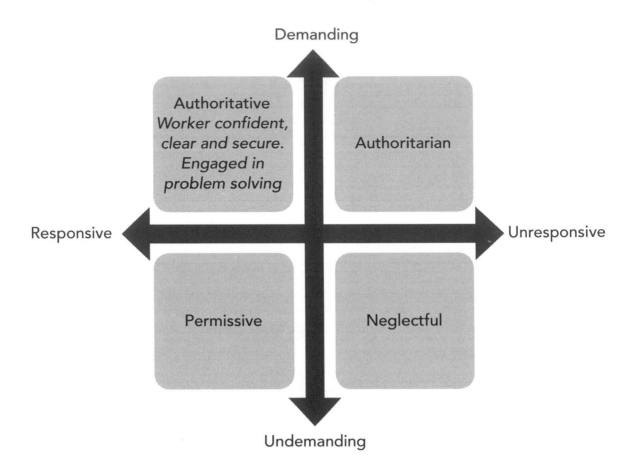

Figure 4.1: Supervisory style. Reprinted with permission from Wonnacott J (2012) *Mastering Social Work Supervision.* **London: JKP**

Being an authoritative supervisor requires an understanding of power, as well as being able to use authority. French and Raven (1959), usefully summarised in Gast and Patmore (2012), identified several forms of power.

1. **Legitimate positional power** – given by organisations which are recognised by the society/culture within which people live. Examples in the context of the UK include the Prime Minister, the head teacher, the registered manager.

2. **Reward power** – power that is able to reward others. This might be, but does not always have to be, linked to a financial gain. The growth of social online networks such as LinkedIn are examples of reward power. People band together with others in the expectation that their association may be mutually beneficial.

3. **Coercive power** – is when others do as they are told because they fear the power of another. It may happen in organisations where punitive sanctions are put in place. The school system is adopting this approach in relation to fining parents whose children are absent during term time.

4. **Expert power** – where people's qualifications put them in a different relationship with others. Examiners for children's activities will usually require a level of expert power to judge dance or music examinations for example. Expert power may come to the fore in certain meetings, for example child protection case conferences will seek to involve people with a range of different expertise.

5. **Referent power** – attributable to individuals, who are often described as charismatic. These tend to be individuals others aspire to be like.

6. **Informational power** – when whoever has access to information holds a level of power. Within early years those practitioners who have a right to access information about others know things that other practitioners may not because they do not have the same access to information, e.g. details of child protection plans or decisions from the management committee.

Many forms of power overlap, and while they can be used for mutually beneficial purposes, some are very likely to leave open the possibility of misuse. The expectation within the EYFS of every child having equality of opportunity stresses the importance of practitioners' understanding power and its potential misuse. For example making sure information about and within the provision is written using the languages of the communities living nearby. Or the fact that early years practitioners are likely to have much more specialised knowledge of child development (i.e. expert power) than many parents.

In relation to an understanding of power supervisors need to be sufficiently self-aware about how they are perceived and the impact their actions may have on others, because of the relative status they hold in society and particularly within their local community.

Most of the thinking in this chapter about authoritative supervision is going to focus on authority. Again, power and authority overlap. Some authority is acquired through the role of supervisor; by being the manager of another practitioner (as the initial definition of supervision makes clear). The ambition of an authoritative supervisor is to work collaboratively and empower practitioners. Nevertheless there may be occasions when swift decision making is required and the supervisor, because of their role, may be required to act decisively, for example to protect a child.

Other elements of authority combine in the effective supervisor. Supervisors have to be able to understand how they make use of their personal power, using their own assertiveness appropriately and confidently to bring an element of personal authority to their working life. If they are to gain the trust of their supervisees supervisors need to be viewed as professionals with integrity; this arises from how they use their personal authority in carrying out aspects of their role.

It is also important when working in a professional role that supervisors have comparable professional knowledge as their supervisees. They need to be able to facilitate informed decision making and therefore the ability to act using professional authority or, equally importantly, to recognise when they have reached the limits of such knowledge. An example of appropriately seeking additional professional knowledge in an authoritative manner might be recognising when the knowledge of a medical practitioner may be required to develop a child's learning journey because the child has specific medical needs, which no one in the provision has previous knowledge or experience of, for example cystic fibrosis, where the child may require specific exercises or dietary needs that differ from other children in the provision or with the same condition.

The authoritative supervisor knows the importance of collaboration; supervisors working to empower their supervisees in the process of engaging effectively and affectively with the task (in this case providing high quality services to children). This links to the concept of reflective practice to encourage development in children within early years settings as outlined by Marbina *et al* (2010). Both Wonnacott (2013) and Marbina *et al* (2010) emphasise the importance of reflection; thinking about the impact of the task on the child as well as the practitioner's role and impact of their work on them. In order to make the child's learning journey a realistic concept, practitioners need to understand how they approach this child in particular, using their past experiences and also their knowledge and observations about this unique child. The supervisor's role is to facilitate this reflective space for the practitioner to bring their knowledge, observations of the child and self-awareness, and to challenge, if required, the activities or actions required to improve the outcomes for the child. For example, as well as playing outside using their gross motor skills children should be encouraged in choosing a story to be read aloud so that they develop some of their executive functioning abilities, such as making choices and listening to others.

As managers, authoritative supervisors should be clear about the roles and tasks they give their supervisees, ensuring practitioners have the skills or the opportunity to acquire knowledge. It is also important that the supervisor questions and challenges the practitioner about the quality of their practice, having high expectations of what they can achieve. Equally, they remain alert to the emotional needs of their supervisees. These important features of authoritative supervision have already been introduced in previous chapters.

Using the ideas outlined here practitioners should begin to picture their ideal authoritative supervisor. Very often the ideas about 'good' or 'poor' supervisors come from our previous experiences of supervision or being managed in other work experiences.

Thinking point

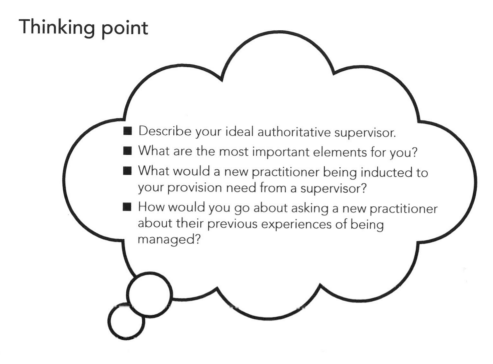

- Describe your ideal authoritative supervisor.
- What are the most important elements for you?
- What would a new practitioner being inducted to your provision need from a supervisor?
- How would you go about asking a new practitioner about their previous experiences of being managed?

Leading on from this thinking point you may be beginning to recognise that practitioners may need different things from supervision depending on their individual circumstances. How do effective authoritative supervisors ensure supervision meets the unique needs of each practitioner? The model used in this guide stresses the importance of building relationships between supervisor and supervisee. Supervisors will be assessing supervisee's competence and forming a view about how much direction the supervisee requires. The aim is to increase professional competence. Figures 4.2 and 4.3 summarise the steps on the journey of professional development and increasing the capacity to act autonomously.

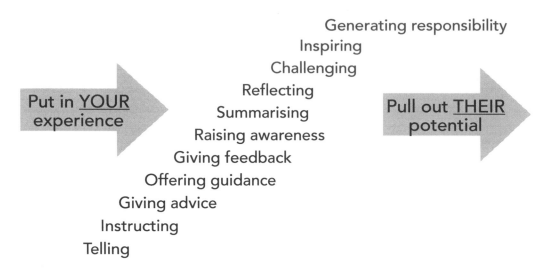

Put in YOUR experience

Generating responsibility
Inspiring
Challenging
Reflecting
Summarising
Raising awareness
Giving feedback
Offering guidance
Giving advice
Instructing
Telling

Pull out THEIR potential

Figure 4.2: Adapted from Downey M (2003) *Effective Coaching: Lessons from the coach's coach* **(2nd edition). London: Cengage Learning**

Supervisory needs			
Directing ■ Structure ■ Information ■ Teaching ■ Constructive and regular feedback ■ Encouragement	**Mentoring** ■ Freedom to test out ■ Space to learn from mistakes ■ Reflection on realities and constraints	**Coaching** ■ Freedom to initiate ■ Further professional development ■ To be stretched and challenged ■ Danger – boredom	**Delegating** ■ To be given wider responsibility ■ To have their experience utilised ■ Less frequent supervision ■ Consults with other professionals

Figure 4.3: Supervisory needs

Effective relationships incorporate trust and respect for each other. Neither of these things are guaranteed to be in place. Trust will be developed depending on how supervisors and supervisees work together and whether the supervisor does what they have told the supervisee they will. If one party repeatedly alters the arrangement for supervision for example, it will not be possible to build trust up within the relationship as the other person will not feel valued.

In the context of professional conversations the terms of that conversation should be clarified including, but not limited to, how disagreements get sorted out. In the pro-forma of a supervision agreement which follows, these points are raised under the section of the form entitled 'Making supervision work'. It is also important to clarify how that authority is used. Misuse of power is always unacceptable and codes of conduct and expectations of each other become essential in conveying trust and respect. The 4x4x4 model used here sees a supervision agreement as an essential component of effective supervision. Agreeing the terms of supervision is a process that facilitates the development of a relationship within supervision. Before a written agreement is signed, a discussion is needed about the elements which are personal to the two people involved. While there is a template included within this guide it should never be used proscriptively or in advance of the conversation taking place between a supervisor and a supervisee. The pitfall, especially once supervision becomes audited, is that the supervision agreement becomes a tick box exercise and at worst filled in by a supervisor without any reference to the supervisee.

There are five steps to establishing an effective working agreement for supervision, firstly establishing why there is a need for supervision. Usually this is a requirement and in early years settings it is now a statutory requirement, therefore there is a non-negotiable element to this.

However, once that is established the process of engaging practitioners in the process begins. The supervisor may think about how to engage with the practitioner as their supervisee and what is required to build a working relationship together, what each side requires for this to be meaningful to them. This does also need to acknowledge the ambivalence they both may be feeling about being in this position. This is especially the situation during the transition in early years to accommodate the changed expectation. Many practitioners will have gone years without being expected to receive supervision, so to suddenly be told they have to have it, and potentially from a newer member of staff arriving in the provision, might lead to resentment if not managed proactively. There could be tensions around experience and qualification that need to be spoken about before meaningful commitment takes place.

The process of writing an agreement, even if a pro-forma for the provision is used, will take a few meetings between supervisor and supervisee to enable each party to express their views having had time to think them through. Significantly, for the agreement to be effective it has to be a document that each party knows about and can reference whenever they need to as part of making supervision effective. The agreement has to live up to its descriptor; a process of agreeing how two people decide they are going to work together with shared aims and expectations which they have had the opportunity to discuss with each other and know they can change should they need to.

1. **Establishing the mandate**
2. **Engaging with the supervisee**
3. **Acknowledging ambivalence**
4. **The written agreement**
5. **Reviewing the agreement**

Supervisory working alliance
The value of a written agreement lies less in the paperwork than in the process by which it has been established

Figure 4.4: Developing the supervisory agreement. Reprinted with permission from Wonnacott J (2014) *Developing and Supporting Staff Supervision Training Pack*. **Brighton: Pavilion Publishing & Media**

The pro-forma that follows is therefore offered as a guide, with the expectation that every supervisor will write a different agreement with each supervisee and that the agreement will be reviewed and changed as the supervisory relationship matures.

SAMPLE SUPERVISION AGREEMENT

Supervision Agreement

Agreement between.. **and** ....

This agreement is designed to be a working tool to underpin the development and maintenance of a good supervisory relationship. The agreement should be:

■ completed at the start of a new supervisory relationship

■ reviewed at least once a year.

The expectations of the provision regarding supervision are set out within the supervision policy, are non-negotiable and provide the framework for this agreement.

The effectiveness of the supervision agreement depends upon the quality of conversation between the supervisor and supervisee, and it is very important that this document provides a foundation for discussion. It should be completed at the conclusion of an exploration of the issues and not become a form filling exercise.

Practical Arrangements

Frequency of one-to-one supervision ....

Duration ....

Venue ....

Arrangements if either party needs to cancel ....

....

Availability of the supervisor for ad hoc discussions between sessions will be

....

Content

The process for agreeing the agenda will be ....

....

Preparation for supervision will include ....

....

....

Particular priority areas to be discussed regularly ....

....

....

Making Supervision Work

What does the supervisee bring to this relationship (e.g. previous work experience, experience of being supervised, preferred learning style)? ....

....

....

....

What are the supervisee's expectations of the supervisor? ....

....

....

....

What are the supervisor's expectations of the supervisee? ....

....

....

....

Are there any factors to acknowledge as relevant to the development of the supervisory relationship (e.g. race, culture, gender, sexual orientation, impairment, including learning difficulties)?

....

....

....

Agreed 'permissions' e.g. It is OK for the supervisor not to know all the answers/for the supervisee to say they are stuck, etc. ....

....

....

....

How will we recognise when the supervisory relationship is not working effectively?

....

....

....

What methods will be used to resolve any difficulties in working together?

....

....

....

Any other relevant issues for this agreement?

....

....

....

Recording

Any decisions made in formal or informal supervision about a child will be recorded on the child's record. Responsibility for this lies with

....

....

The content of one-to-one supervision sessions regarding the development and support needs of the supervisee will be recorded, agreed by both parties and placed in the supervisee's file. Responsibility for this lies with

....

....

Date agreement due to be reviewed:

Signed:

Supervisor:

Supervisee:

Date:

Thinking point

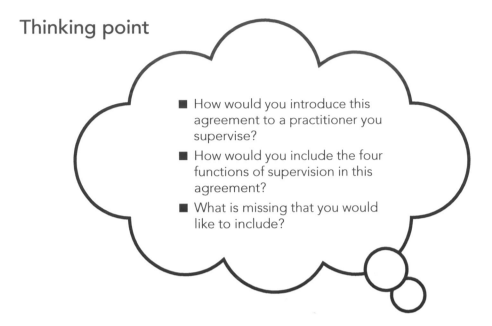

- How would you introduce this agreement to a practitioner you supervise?
- How would you include the four functions of supervision in this agreement?
- What is missing that you would like to include?

Recording supervision

Amidst much debate among early years practitioners, the writers of this guide (in the absence of clarity elsewhere) are encouraging the good practice of recording separately what is discussed in supervision about each child, and what is recorded that relates to the practitioner. Each provider has to think through and provide policies about how information will be collected and for what purposes it will be stored. Practitioner's employment records should be stored confidentially and practitioners should be confident that whatever they discuss in supervision is not available to their peers. They should also be aware of under what circumstances information from their supervision record may be shared elsewhere, e.g. if there was a capability issue. As part of the agreement there needs to be recognition that supervision records form part of the employee record. Supervisees are given a copy of what has been recorded about them from supervision and are encouraged to read them and raise it with their supervisor if they feel the recording is an inaccurate account of their discussion.

Similarly where there are child protection concerns or issues about a child's development then the provision has to have clear, confidential arrangements for the storage of those records. Part of the decision making process in the supervisory meeting should include how and when the information will be shared with the parent(s) of the child. An important task for each provider is to decide which information is kept with the 'Child's Journey' (i.e. the daily record of what the child is doing that is freely available within the provision) and which in the child's confidential file. This policy will need to link to the supervisory policy so that practitioners and supervisors are clear what needs to be recorded where.

Thinking point

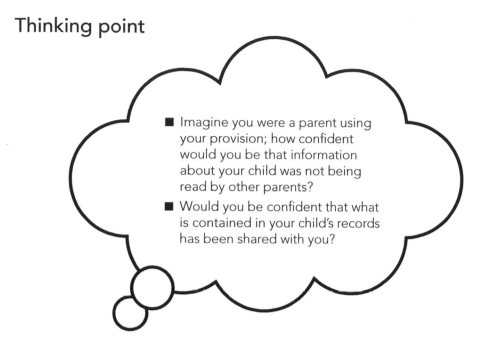

■ Imagine you were a parent using your provision; how confident would you be that information about your child was not being read by other parents?

■ Would you be confident that what is contained in your child's records has been shared with you?

Included here are ideas about a structure for recording supervision; they give a framework that could be used as an agenda. However, effective supervision relies on the negotiation between two people and their ability to trust one another in carrying out the tasks expected of their roles. Therefore any pro-forma should be flexible and should be seen as a tool to be adapted.

SAMPLE SUPERVISION RECORD

Supervision Record

Supervisee

Date

Supervisor

Agenda item	Summary of discussion	Decisions/ actions	Responsible person	Timescale
Issues relating to staff development E.g. feedback from training, progress in respect of continuing professional development.				
Issues relating to practitioner support E.g. sickness/annual leave, any current stressors or issues relating to practitioner well-being (including workload review). Reasonable adjustments under Equalities Act if required.				

Agenda item	Summary of discussion	Decisions/ actions	Responsible person	Timescale
Issues relating to professional practice and provider requirements E.g. impact of any new policies/procedures/ organisational expectations. Consideration of what has worked well in relation to practice. Any issues relating to quality of practice/ performance.				
Any other issues				

A copy to be given to supervisee and a copy retained and filed securely by the supervisor.

Signed: supervisor — Date

Signed: supervisee — Date

SAMPLE CHILD RECORD SHEET

Supervision Record

Child	
Supervisee	Supervisor
Date	

Agenda item	Summary of discussion		Decisions/ actions	Responsible person	Timescale
	Experience/information discussed (seeing)	Reflections (feelings)			

Agenda item	Summary of discussion	Decisions/ actions	Responsible person	Timescale
Analysis (how understanding of the issues was reached – thinking)				
Action plan – (what needs doing?)				
Signed: supervisor	Date	Copy retained and filed securely by the supervisor on child's record.		
Signed: supervisee	Date			

Thinking point

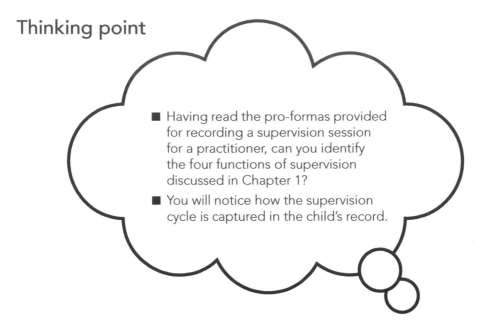

- Having read the pro-formas provided for recording a supervision session for a practitioner, can you identify the four functions of supervision discussed in Chapter 1?
- You will notice how the supervision cycle is captured in the child's record.

Using the concept of the child's journey helps to explain the purpose of the separate processes of recording. Supervision records should show 'the working out' of why decisions about children or practitioners are made. Historically, public organisations have been criticised for not explaining why they do what they do. This lack of transparency has promoted a sense of secrecy and exclusion, often unintentionally. A test that is useful in identifying what needs to be recorded is: if I were a stranger picking up these records would I understand why the decisions were made, can I follow how this child made progress and 'journeyed' through the provision?

The authoritative supervisor builds relationships with supervisees which take account of power and authority and understands how they may be used or abused in supervision. The authoritative supervisor uses their emotional intelligence effectively in their relationships with practitioners. The concept of authoritative supervisory practice has offered a structure in this chapter to introduce the importance of developing a working agreement between supervisor and supervisee. The agreement needs to be more than a document that is filed away for an audit process, it is a key tool in making an effective supervisory relationship. Accurate recording has also been highlighted as it tells the story of how children and practitioners develop in their respective learning journeys. This chapter concludes the core components of supervision. The next chapter explores some of the issues particular to making supervision effective in early years settings.

Chapter 5: What are the issues when implementing supervision for early years providers?

Introduction

This chapter maps the expectations and principles underpinning the framework for the Early Years Foundation Stage (EYFS) (Department for Education, 2014) and links them with supervisory practice. It will explore the recurring challenges arising in implementing the statutory requirement of supervision. Using composite examples of different types of provider, a range of issues are explored. These are the frequently occurring questions that trainers may face in delivering the programme. It is also intended to help providers reach solutions which work for them.

Issues for early years providers

The EYFS covers a wide range of providers, but in this chapter there is a focus on issues that could arise for childminders where they need to supervise practitioners, committee run community preschools and privately owned nurseries. Case material is used to initiate debate about the issues that could arise when thinking about implementing supervision effectively. While not every situation will be catered for, the expectation is that the ideas and processes will assist early years practitioners to think through the implications of similar issues they could encounter within their own settings.

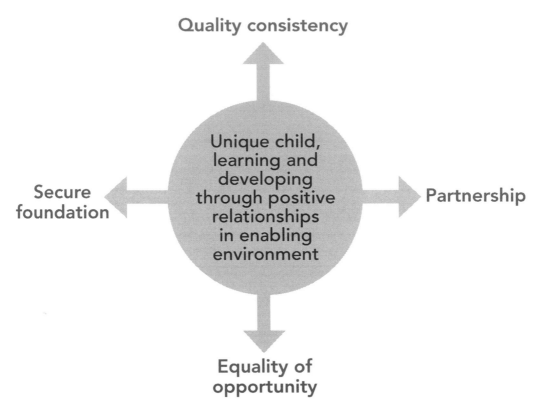

Figure 5.1: Mapping principles of EYFS

In discussing the challenges of implementing supervision and how it could be overcome we will return to this diagram first introduced in chapter 1. This framework will be used to explain how the supervision model presented in this manual can be used to strengthen the principles of the EYFS framework.

Childminders

Childminders are required to be supervisors when they employ assistants to allow them to look after more children.

Case example – Jenny and Sara

Jenny is a very experienced childminder who has been looking after children for the past 15 years. She knows her families well, as they all live on the same estate. She has an assistant to help her every afternoon as she has children who come to her after school. Sara is the daughter of one of Jenny's friends. Sara works in a café in the mornings, and is gaining work experience as she wants to go to college to train as a teacher. Sara is very lively and seems to have an excellent social life. She is quite often tired during the day and her boyfriend, Ben, frequently arrives early to pick her up at the end of the afternoon. Parents are beginning to comment that he is hanging around outside Jenny's house.

What could be the issues raised by this example? Reputation is very important and how childminders are perceived by their local community will affect their business. For childminders, their home is usually their place of work and managing the boundary between work and home has to be a constant area of vigilance for them. Having people 'hanging around', however innocently, affects how they are perceived. If parents are feeling uncomfortable approaching Jenny's house because Ben is loitering outside this becomes a business issue for Jenny. It undermines Jenny's ability to make partnerships with parents if they feel wary of collecting the children.

Thinking point

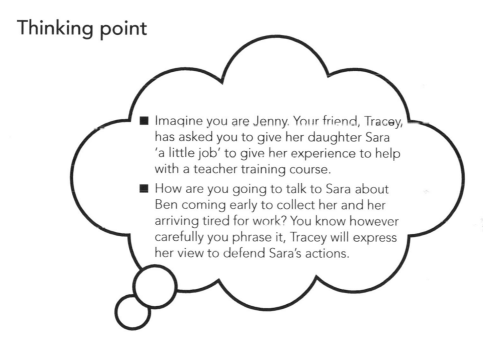

- Imagine you are Jenny. Your friend, Tracey, has asked you to give her daughter Sara 'a little job' to give her experience to help with a teacher training course.
- How are you going to talk to Sara about Ben coming early to collect her and her arriving tired for work? You know however carefully you phrase it, Tracey will express her view to defend Sara's actions.

Childminders and other community based groups are often valued by their local communities because of the close relationship they have with people living nearby. They need to balance their personal and professional relationships alongside their statutory responsibilities. They also have to safeguard the children they are looking after. These are both areas where practitioners may need support. Safeguarding involves both providing safe everyday care, including safe practitioners, and also identifying when a child is at risk of abuse or neglect.

Practitioners need to be proactive in contacting children's social care or the police to make a child protection referral (Department for Education, 2014, para. 3.2 & 3.3) if and when the occasion arises. Knowing that the practitioners they employ are competent and confident in using this professional authority is essential for childminders (and nursery owners/managers) in maintaining professional credibility and providing good quality consistent care.

Jenny needs to know that Sara is alert when she is looking after the children, that she is responsive to their needs and able to prioritise the children over her social life and ignore Ben's presence outside the house. Jenny also has to manage Ben's presence to ensure that he is not putting parents off or affecting how she is being perceived. She needs to ensure that Sara understands these issues and suggests she asks Ben to arrive later or to meet her away from Jenny's house.

In order to tackle these issues effectively, Jenny needs to make sure she has time and a space where she can speak to Sara so that issues related to equality of opportunity for both Sara and the children can be discussed sensitively.

The concept of supervision as a professional conversation stresses both its importance and also its link with the professional task for which the practitioner is being paid. Therefore supervision becomes fundamental to the expectations of the practitioner's work and is an issue raised in our final thoughts. Funding the additional costs of supervision needs further working out. There are financial implications for providing good supervision both in terms of paying practitioners' for their time and additional hire costs of venues suitable for supervision. In many settings, practitioners are paid for their face-to-face contact with children and there are ratios of numbers of children to numbers of staff that must be adhered to (Department for Education, 2014, para. 3.30 - 3.39). Therefore, providing time and space for two practitioners to be away from face-to-face contact in order to ensure the supervision requirement is met will have financial implications which may be a barrier to implementation. Paying practitioners for their skills is an issue that has already been raised with the government in relation to their plans to increase funded childcare places (Adams & Mason, 2015). Financing this time and space may also be an issue for Jenny and could have implications in the fees she charges parents.

Community-based preschools

There are many issues around the governance of preschools (Wonnacott 2013). Preschools often exist as charitable organisations run by a committee with oversight of trustees. Because they are heavily reliant on volunteers to run the committee and because often the volunteers are parents using the preschool for their childcare, there are issues about skills, available time and understanding of the context. Additionally the committee is likely to change every year. In some situations the preschools may be sharing the premises with other organisations, e.g. in local village or church halls.

The case example of Hedgehogs Preschool used in Chapter 2 allows discussion of the kind of issues which face community based and committee run provisions. As a reminder:

Case example – Hedgehogs Preschool

Hedgehogs Preschool is situated in a small rural community and has a very good reputation with local parents, and the most recent Ofsted inspection gave it a 'good' grade. The manager of the preschool lives in the village, as do many of the practitioners, and they tend to socialise both within the practitioner group and with parents in the village outside preschool hours. Practitioners are usually recruited by word of mouth and the majority of the team have worked at the preschool for over five years. The administration for the preschool has been undertaken by parent volunteers but lately the main volunteer has left as she has got a permanent job elsewhere. The preschool has recently recruited two new practitioners from outside the area and one of them has been commenting that a lot of attention is paid to one particular child, Maya, by Hannah, one of the supervisors. Hannah is a popular practitioner and the new practitioner has been reassured that this is because Hannah is a friend of Maya's mother. The team have commented that the two new practitioners do not seem to fit in very well and are very rigid in their ideas about childcare practice.

There is clearly an issue relating to equality of opportunity (Department for Education, 2014, para. 3). How do community based organisations make sure that they are open to all in the local community? In this example Hannah is a friend of Maya's mother. It does not appear uncommon, from the authors' experience, for children to be known by or related to practitioners. Protecting the setting from accusations of favouritism is important in order to meet the expectation of offering equality of opportunity, tailoring the child's journey to them uniquely and evidencing that each child is being given the optimum environment in which they can learn and develop (Department for Education, 2014, para. 3-6). Supervision is a process by which these issues can be explored and discussed. However, to be effective there will need to be a context and culture within the preschool reinforcing those expectations, e.g. policies, welcoming packs and leaflets explaining how the preschool works for parents and carers, and induction processes for practitioners and children (partnership working and quality and consistency).

Thinking point

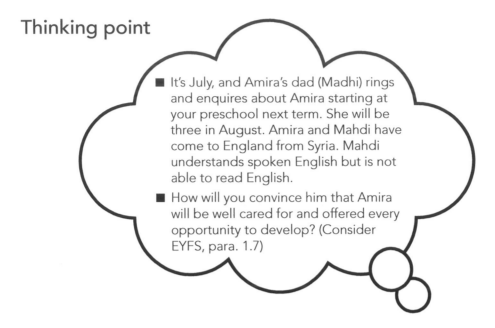

- It's July, and Amira's dad (Madhi) rings and enquires about Amira starting at your preschool next term. She will be three in August. Amira and Mahdi have come to England from Syria. Mahdi understands spoken English but is not able to read English.

- How will you convince him that Amira will be well cared for and offered every opportunity to develop? (Consider EYFS, para. 1.7)

Nursery settings

Many of the issues already covered are also equally pertinent for nursery settings. The positive relationships practitioners make within the provision and outside in the community all affect the success of the business.

Where the owner is effectively the manager too they may find themselves in a similar position to other managers at the top of a hierarchy. The need for reflection and challenge is still required but an issue commonly arising is about making professional relationships with business competitors. Co-operating on a peer consultation model as suggested later may be harder in the context of business rivalry. This is especially true because the success of the peer consultative process requires a degree of trust in each other. Where there are more children requiring places than are available locally it may be easier to work in partnership, than when there is competition to attract children to places. The authors as business owners themselves have found unexpected benefits from collaboration.

Confidentiality

Confidentiality is a challenge in confined spaces especially when sharing facilities with other organisations. The expectation in EYFS is that:

'Providers must also ensure that there is an area where staff may talk to parents and/or carers confidentially, as well as an area in group settings for staff to take breaks away from areas being used by children.'

(Department for Education, 2014, para. 3.61)

It is the authors' view that a confidential space is required for supervision to be able to occur out of the sight and hearing of children, parents and other practitioners. Equally, that the recording of what is said in supervision should be stored confidentially in the practitioner's file and confidentially on each child's record so that it cannot be accessed by anyone unauthorised to do so. It is not clear from the Hedgehogs Preschool example how well that ethos was being put into practice as the culture was one of administration being done by a parent volunteer.

In so-called 'pack away' provisions where facilities are hired for the duration of the children's sessions, confidential space may be unavailable. At a pragmatic level this may mean supervision takes place in practitioners' or supervisors' homes. Thinking about confidentiality, the expectations of supervision and how a supervision agreement is used to reinforce the boundaries of these meetings all require consideration beforehand. How will any power imbalance be affected by whose home is used, how will other people in the home be protected from the discussion and not made a party to them? Preserving confidentiality, including how and where records are stored, is important for developing and maintaining trusting relationships.

Allied to issues of confidentiality are considerations about the physical space in which supervision takes place. Agile working is increasingly expected by contemporary workplaces (Cain, 2011). Commonly referred to as 'hot desking', the idea is that workers can work anywhere and do not require their own personalised space in which to work. Therefore the space workers, certainly in the public sector, have been given to work in has been reduced. This is a paradox at present; there is an expectation of increasingly high professional standards without a recognition of the need for physical space to accomplish processes such as professional conversations and meetings in confidential spaces. Although this concept of agile working is not as commonly used in early years settings, the significance of space for the supervisory task does require separate consideration. Historically, preschool, play groups and community centres offering childcare have provided rooms for the children and their activities but very little or no additional space for confidential conversations such as the EYFS is now stipulating. As the administrative expectations have increased there are issues about the physical space within the provision to get the tasks done.

Thinking point

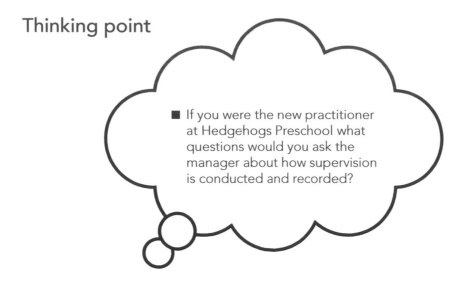

■ If you were the new practitioner at Hedgehogs Preschool what questions would you ask the manager about how supervision is conducted and recorded?

Committees

The other two main issues arising in a preschool context are associated with one another. One is how practitioners who work closely within their communities, and are accountable to a changing group of parents, are able to maintain their professionalism. The second is the role of the preschool committee chair. The boundaries between parent, parent helper/volunteer, committee member and practitioner can get very blurred in small communities. There may be only one provider in a village. Becoming a parent while maintaining a career in education may make working in the local community preschool attractive. It fits with school hours and gives parents similar holidays. Managing the boundary between being the parent of a child in the preschool (or knowing other parents of the preschool socially because your older children are together in the village school) and working in the preschool has to be carefully managed so that everyone else in the community continues to trust in the integrity of the preschool. These issues require discussion during supervision. Clarifying personal and professional relationships is a key part of establishing an effective supervision agreement.

Thinking point

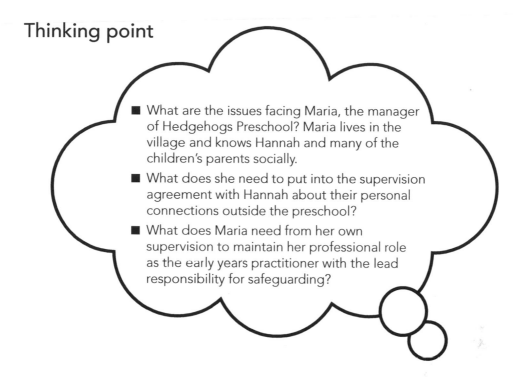

- What are the issues facing Maria, the manager of Hedgehogs Preschool? Maria lives in the village and knows Hannah and many of the children's parents socially.
- What does she need to put into the supervision agreement with Hannah about their personal connections outside the preschool?
- What does Maria need from her own supervision to maintain her professional role as the early years practitioner with the lead responsibility for safeguarding?

The role of the committee, who are likely to also be parents of the children in the provision, may further blur accountability issues. These are important areas of discussion for providers to establish clear policies and procedures which clarify the level and limits of responsibility. The committee may not be able to provide guidance around the professional nature of the task of running the preschool. There needs to be clear role definitions about what is and isn't important for committee members to know.

The role of the preschool committee chair needs to be carefully defined and the limits of confidentiality clarified. Child protection issues should be kept confidential to those with professional responsibility for ensuring children are safeguarded. Similarly if there are specific developmental issues, the child should not be identifiable to committee members even if the particular issues may require discussion in the committee meetings e.g. how to afford specific equipment. Preschool committee chairs may feel they need to know about and to attend child protection case conferences in their role as the preschool committee chair. Preschool managers are encouraged to challenge and ask what purpose the chair's attendance has for the child and family. The purpose of the child protection conference is to make a child protection plan. How will the chair's role contribute to a child protection plan?

It is also important to emphasise the confidential nature of the information shared in a child protection conference. Committee chairs do not need to know identifying detail about children as long as the providers are confident in their decision making and capable of taking the actions they need to. It is in this area that supervision has a function in clarifying the accountabilities for the decision making. The preschool manager is the early years professional with the responsibility for ensuring the professional task is carried out within the expectations of the EYFS framework. The role of the preschool committee chair is to ensure the governance functions are met and this does include a general oversight of the running of the preschool. It is important that the boundaries of each role are discussed and recorded in an agreement about how each party understands their role.

These matters around supervision have to be explicitly discussed in order for the trust in supervision to be exercised effectively. Withholding information undermines supervision as an effective tool in practitioner development.

It is equally important that the committee understands its responsibility for maintaining the integrity of the preschool and that members are not seen gossiping outside about preschool matters. Depending on the location and size of the provision, finding volunteers to take the roles is challenging enough without setting criteria about their eligibility. Whether committee members have a professional grasp of the issues in early years settings varies. Therefore the person who becomes the chair also affects the quality of the oversight of the preschool. Preschool managers have learnt to become self-reliant in terms of managing themselves and the practitioners in the provision adjusting to an unpredictable quality of management. However, improving practice and responding to changing environments while motivating others is challenging without good emotional support and stimulation, so it is important that good supervision is provided to managers as well as practitioners.

Whether the chair of the preschool is the best person to supervise the manager, although clearly the preschool manager is accountable to the chair, has to be clearly thought through. It is unlikely that they will hold the role long term and they may not have professional skills or expertise relevant to developing the practitioners in the post. An adaptation of the model for supervision may become necessary so that the accountability issues are discussed with the preschool committee chair and the other functions of supervision (specifically professional development, management of the task and emotional support) are offered perhaps using a peer/group consultation model with other preschool managers.

In current contexts expanding the role of the local authority early years adviser to facilitate such consultative groups is looking unlikely as their role and remit is reduced. However, this could perhaps be reviewed and considered. Early years advisers may be well placed to have a lead role in these developments, as they often have relevant experience of working as early years practitioners as well as the experience of receiving/delivering supervision.

It may be that formal alliances with negotiated agreements about how professional matters are conducted are built between neighbouring preschools. The supervision cycle used here is the universal model proposed for adult learning and development including supervision (Davys & Beddoe, 2010). The templates in the previous chapter allow for adaptation about which topics require discussion with the preschool chair (e.g. staffing) and which will be the focus of a peer arrangement, e.g. professional development or managing the environment to facilitate the optimal development of children using the provision.

Perhaps there will be a need for two agreements rather than one which clarify the different expectations. One that clarifies the managerial accountabilities to the preschool chair and another with the peer or peer group which is about the development, mediation and emotional support functions of supervision around the professional task. It is important to consider how conflict between the two roles will be mediated and whether a neutral third party could be used if there are irreconcilable differences of opinion about professional/managerial decision making. However, what is essential is that the process is explicitly contracted and agreed so that all are clear about what should be discussed where, and what responsibilities may be delegated to others.

To stress the importance of these professional conversations, which are designed to promote professional development, the time and space should be paid for and seen as part of the manager's work.

Business versus ethical issues

Where the value base of practitioners and the EYFS framework are congruent with each other this increases the likelihood of effective outcomes for children. Owners running nurseries for business profit without necessarily understanding the professional implications in the guidance may struggle with understanding why supervisory time is so essential to the task. It might be helpful for managers to take owners through some of the stakeholder benefits covered in the earlier chapters.

Maintaining healthy, professional relationships

Effective management of the professional relationships within early years provision is an ongoing challenge. Highlighted from the nursery reviews (Plymouth Safeguarding Children Board, 2010; Birmingham Safeguarding Children Board, 2012) and summarised by Wonnacott (2013), there are two issues. The first is about building confidence in practitioners to notice and be sufficiently curious and concerned about colleagues' behaviour. The second is then to ensure managers or the overseeing committees/owners are sufficiently approachable and capable of hearing what is making practitioners uneasy. These are both essential to protect children from abuse within early years settings. Wonnacott states that the culture within the provision needs to emphasise a strong focus on safety in order for practitioners to feel able to speak up and be heard. This observation builds on Nutbrown's review into early years settings highlighting concerns about practitioners' confidence in their knowledge base and professional assertiveness (Nutbrown, 2012).

Thinking point

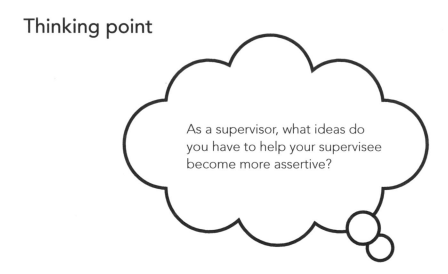

As a supervisor, what ideas do you have to help your supervisee become more assertive?

Maintaining professional relationships and managing differences of opinion and views are essential in creating enabling environments for children. It is also required to ensure equality of opportunity. Working effectively with diverse communities and facilitating children's development whatever their needs, requires discussions amongst practitioners to build skills and knowledge and challenge practice which may be discriminatory. These factors have been picked up and reinforced in the EYFS expectation that supervision:

'…fosters a culture of mutual support, teamwork and continuous improvement which encourages the confidential discussion of sensitive issues.'
(Department for Education, 2014, para. 3.19)

Therefore expectations are in place that practitioners should develop the habit of discussing their own and other people's practice and supervision is the place to have these professional conversations. Supervisors are well placed to identify commonly arising issues that may need addressing throughout the setting and to decide whether they should be raised in team meetings or as individual performance issues. It is the supervisor's responsibility to hold the boundaries of supervision as a professional conversation that discusses practice issues and to make sure that gossip about people is not tolerated.

Working in early years is a career that attracts many young people. Young women looking for their first job like the idea of working with children. It is a comparatively accessible profession, as although there is an option of a university entrance, it is not a prerequisite as it is for other careers. Some entrants to the early years workforce may therefore still be maturing in terms of their own development and establishing their own identity. For example understanding the boundaries between what was acceptable at school when commenting on social media and what is acceptable now they are in a professional role. This issue will need ongoing and at times close management.

Professional boundaries are complicated by relationships practitioners may have with friends living locally outside the provision. It may be necessary to 'defriend' parents on social media while their children are using the provision. Guidance around use of social media will be part of the policies within each provision. However practitioners will need to understand why these boundaries are necessary, in order to comply with this. Managers need to ensure they have systems of overseeing practitioners and encouraging whistleblowing to ensure practice is not defensive, and that younger or less confident practitioners who witness bad practice are facilitated in exploring what they have seen (for example how Joanne was helped to explore what she meant by 'probably nothing' in Chapter 2). All these processes are subjects which can be raised within the relationship a supervisor and supervisee create and are encouraged by the frank discussion which form part of negotiating a supervision agreement together.

Thinking point

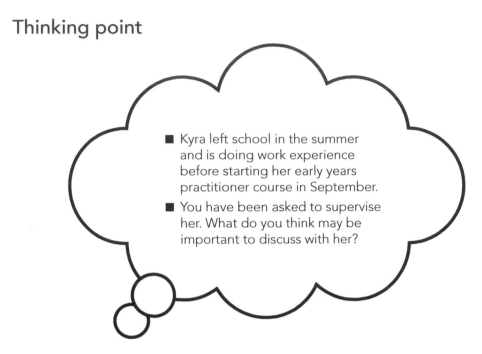

- Kyra left school in the summer and is doing work experience before starting her early years practitioner course in September.
- You have been asked to supervise her. What do you think may be important to discuss with her?

There are a number of issues in getting supervision established within the range of early years providers. This chapter has discussed the regularly emerging issues such as time, space, confidentiality and roles by focusing on childminding, preschools and privately run nurseries. The following chapter will look at how the culture of supervision gets taken on by the management and leadership team to embed the process successfully.

Chapter 6: Establishing a culture of supervision

Introduction

Supervision is a new concept to early years providers; it was first introduced in the guidance issued in 2012. Early years providers must now provide supervision to practitioners and volunteers (Department for Education, 2014). The statutory expectation builds on the advisory 'should' used in the guidance previous to 2012. For supervision to be effective there needs to be a culture within each provision that reinforces and builds on expectations about supervision. This chapter looks at how to build a culture in which effective supervision can flourish. Using the appreciative inquiry framework of what is working well and how it can be improved, tools are provided to audit supervisory practice and ideas for establishing the culture effectively.

How supervision is essential to safe practice

Supervision as outlined in Chapter 1 is part of maintaining safe practices within the setting. In thinking about the importance of supervision and establishing a culture of supervision it is worth restating some of the observations from earlier chapters. In Chapter 2 the impact of supervision on the key stakeholders was investigated. This is the heart of the 4x4x4 model, the people who benefit from effective supervision. The benefits to the child emphasised their learning and development stimulated by high quality consistent care provided within an enabling, safe environment. The practitioner developed their own skills, shared their worries about their own or others' practice and was supported in their role to achieve higher standards. For providers the importance of happy children cannot be underestimated, as parents ultimately make decisions about whether they will continue to support the provision determined by their view about the safety and well-being of their child. Therefore, key to the success of the business is keeping children happy by having a safe environment and skilled practitioners.

Supervision becomes part of the method for achieving these aims. In an earlier chapter it was likened to the early warning system. Practitioners should be encouraged to report their observations and their feedback about their own and others' practice in a way that encourages transparency and trust. These are factors that protect children in group environments. Green (2012) summarises the main factors of a safe organisation providing group care to children:

'1 Robust recruitment procedures

2 Written codes of conduct

3 Expectation that practitioners follow codes of conduct

4 Induction and regular training review

5 SUPERVISION, policy and carried out

6 Know about whistle blowing policy and how to use it

7 Prompt and robust action when concerns raised

8 Work closely with multi-disciplinary team colleagues and accept their advice when needed

9 Understand difference between criminal behaviour and what falls outside the code of conduct

10 Follow disciplinary procedures appropriately

11 Ensure procedures and process is fair.'

Green (2012 p.186)

Supervision is one way of making sure practitioners know what is expected of them and that they are adhering to the codes of conduct and policies of the provider. When linked with performance appraisal it becomes a transparent process of developing and improving practitioner competence thereby increasing confidence in parents and others that children are safe, happy and learning.

Thinking point

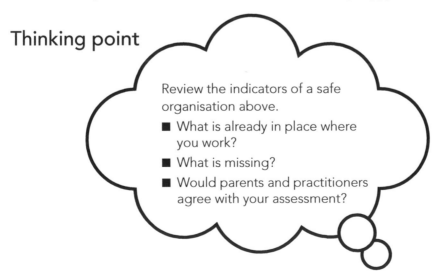

Review the indicators of a safe organisation above.

■ What is already in place where you work?

■ What is missing?

■ Would parents and practitioners agree with your assessment?

Safe organisations provide supervision to and of their staff

Having stated the importance of supervision in safeguarding children, it is imperative that the culture is reinforced by the leadership team in the provision. In thinking about how to establish a culture of supervision in settings where this is an unfamiliar concept Figure 6.1 has been used. It is designed to demonstrate the process of getting supervision embedded into the culture and practice of each provision.

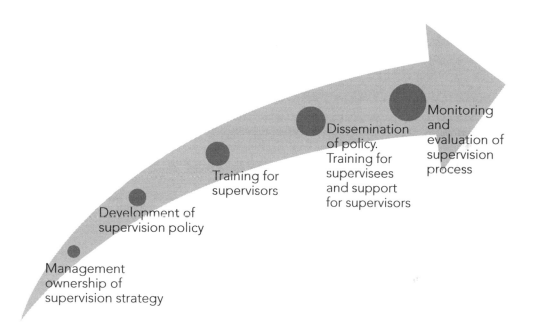

Figure 6.1: Developing a supervision culture

Management ownership of the supervision strategy and developing supervision policy

In previous chapters there has been discussion about some of the challenges presented in making supervision a reality in early years. However it is now a statutory requirement. While acknowledging that there may still remain some resistance, nevertheless supervision has to be part of every early years provision where there is more than a lone practitioner (Department for Education, 2014). Understanding why it has been made a statutory requirement and the explicit link with safer practice and keeping children and practitioners protected begins to shift resistance.

The leadership role requires managers and owners to sell the benefits of supervision within their provision. The importance of supervision being a safe space to reflect on what workers have done well and to think about how to improve. An opportunity to identify learning needs. The space to reflect on the impact working with children can have. This guide provides ideas about how this can be done. However, in order for this to be effective it is helpful to have a policy which makes clear what the leadership see as the purpose and aim of supervision for their particular setting. Below is a template that can be used to begin the process. As with all the templates included in this guide it is intended as a starting point for discussion with the key people who need to make supervision effective in each setting. Like all policies and procedures, none are effective unless they make sense to practitioners in their workplace.

SAMPLE OUTLINE SUPERVISION POLICY

1	Introduction
1.1	*'Providers must put appropriate arrangements in place for the supervision of staff who have contact with children and families. Effective supervision provides support, coaching and training for the practitioner and promotes the interests of children. Supervision should foster a culture of mutual support, teamwork and continuous improvement which encourages the confidential discussion of sensitive issues.'* (Department for Education, 2014, para. 3.19)
1.2	*'Supervision should provide opportunities for staff to:* ■ *discuss any issues – particularly concerning children's development or well-being;* ■ *identify solutions to address issues as they arise; and* ■ *receive coaching to improve their personal effectiveness.'* (Department for Education, 2014, para. 3.20)
1.3	Supervision is a requirement of the Early Years Foundation Stage and this policy is based on the premise that the supervision of practitioners is an integral part of the day-to-day business of our setting. It will occur both formally and in other forums, including informal discussions and group settings, and in all of these forums the process of supervision should be informed by the standards set out within this document.

1.4	[This provision] recognises that:
	■ Supervision of practitioners is integral to the effective delivery of services.
	■ The quality of practitioner supervision impacts on outcomes for children and their families.
	■ The delivery of supervision must be a priority task within the provision.
	■ All practitioners have the right to receive regular formal supervision from supervisors who have received appropriate training and are supported within their supervisory role.
	■ All practitioners [including volunteer/parent helpers?] have a responsibility to participate in supervision and attend formal sessions.
	■ The process of supervision is a shared responsibility; practitioners and their supervisors are expected to contribute to the effectiveness of the process and the provision has a responsibility to facilitate a culture which supports the process.
2	**Scope**
2.1	[To be developed/agreed within the provision depending upon organisational structure.]
3	**Definition – what is supervision?** [To be developed/agreed within the provision but could be based on the definition below.]
3.1	For the purposes of this policy, supervision is defined as a process by which one practitioner is given responsibility by the provision to work with another worker(s) in order to meet certain organisational, professional and personal objectives to therefore promote positive outcomes for service users. The objectives are: ■ Competent, accountable performance (managerial function). ■ Continuing professional development (educational/development function). ■ Personal support (supportive function). ■ Linking the individual to the organisation (mediation function). (Definition adapted from Morrison (2005) *Staff Supervision in Social Care*. Brighton: Pavilion Publishing).
3.2	The process of supervision is supported by the development of a relationship between supervisors and supervisees which provides a safe environment to support the practitioner and facilitate reflection, challenge and critical thinking.

4	**Statement of expectations** [To be developed/agreed within the provision but could be based on the paragraphs below.]
4.1	**The provision will:** ■ Prioritise supervision as an important activity within the service. ■ Ensure that all practitioners who come within the scope of this policy have a named supervisor who also has line management responsibility for their work and welfare. ■ Provide training and ongoing development opportunities for supervisors. ■ Ensure appropriate space is provided for one-to-one meetings. ■ Regularly evaluate the quality of supervision being provided.
4.2	**Supervisors will:** ■ Ensure the delivery of one-to-one supervision sessions at a frequency in line with this policy. ■ Ensure that supervision is recorded in line with the expectations set out within this policy. ■ Ensure that the prime focus of supervision is the quality of service being received by children and families. ■ Use the supervision agreement as the basis for the development of a relationship where supervisees can be supported in their work and to reflect on their practice. ■ Ensure the supervisee is clear about how to raise any concerns about the quality of supervision being received. ■ Use the supervisory process to learn from good practice and give constructive feedback in order to promote professional development. ■ Address performance concerns as they arise and work positively with the supervisee to improve practice. ■ Take responsibility for their personal development as a supervisor and use their own supervision to reflect on their supervisory practice.
4.3	**Supervisees will:** ■ Take responsibility for attending one-to-one supervision or group sessions as set out in their supervision agreement. ■ Prepare adequately for supervision and take an active part in the process. ■ Take responsibility for raising any concerns they may have about the quality of the supervisory relationship with the supervisor or, if this is not possible, the third party named within the supervision agreement.
5	**Method of delivery** [To be developed/agreed within the provision but could be based on the paragraphs below.]

5.1	A relationship between a supervisor and supervisee is fundamental to the supervisory process and supervision will take place in a variety of settings and circumstances.
5.2	One-to-one supervision is at the heart of the process and all staff should receive regular formal one-to-one supervision.
5.3	Ad hoc supervision is the dialogue that takes place between a supervisor and supervisee as the need arises. This should be available to all practitioners but is not a substitute for formal one-to-one supervision. The value of ad hoc supervision is that it is an important way of supporting practitioners, improving performance, keeping pace with change and ensuring that the setting's requirements are met. It should be recorded in line with these procedures.
6	**Frequency** [To be developed/agreed within the provision.]
7	**The supervision agreement**
7.1	The development of a productive supervisory relationship starts with: ■ Clarity about roles and responsibilities and requirements of the provision. ■ Building rapport, understanding each others' perspective and any factors that might affect the process. ■ Acknowledging that effective supervision may not always be comfortable and exploring how power, authority and differences of opinion may be negotiated.
7.2	This process should be captured within the written agreement and it is the responsibility of supervisors to ensure that an agreement is in place for every supervisee using the provision's template. This agreement should be signed by both parties and placed in the supervisee's file.
7.3	The written agreement is a working tool and should be reviewed at least once a year.
8	**Supervision process and content** [To be developed/agreed within the provision but could refer to the four functions of supervision and the use of the supervision cycle.]
9	**Recording supervision** [To be developed/agreed within the provision.]
10	**Monitoring and review** [To be developed/agreed within the provision – but should include a process for obtaining supervisee feedback on the process.]

Thinking point

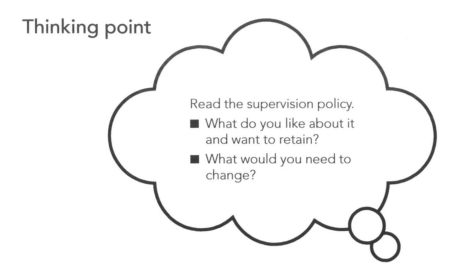

Read the supervision policy.
■ What do you like about it and want to retain?
■ What would you need to change?

Contained within the supervision policy are the various chapters of the guide that define the 4x4x4 model. The definition of supervision is that used in Chapter 1. The rim of the model includes the four aspects of supervision (management, mediation, development and support). The purpose of supervision and expectations about its functions need to be clear within the supervision policy. They should follow through into each agreement between supervisor and supervisee. It is useful if these elements form part of a recording template too as a further reminder of the purpose of having supervision. Therefore, to successfully embed a supervision culture there should be a supervision policy, linking to an agreement and recording template suitable for each provider. The templates are expected to be used flexibly for the specific needs of each practitioner and should reflect the needs of each unique child in the setting.

For supervision to be effective, it is essential that all participants in the process understand why they are having supervision. Expectations on supervisors and supervisees should be explicit with both parties agreeing on how they will make supervision work for them and what to do if it does not. The focus must be on providing services to children that enable them to learn and develop in their own unique way. It may be helpful to reference the overarching principles of EYFS in the policy too.

Alongside the principles of EYFS about improving outcomes for the child is a recognition of the reach of supervision to benefit the people who are at the heart of the 4x4x4 model (Chapter 2). The four stakeholders are also referenced in the policy; the child, the practitioner, the provision, the external partners (families and other agencies the provider works with).

How supervision is going to work, the methods and frequency, will include a discussion about the supervisory cycle from chapter 3. In order to maintain professional development practitioners need opportunities to participate in all four elements of the supervisory cycle; seeing, feeling, thinking and doing. This links the heart of the model to its rim. The more practitioners and supervisors understand about the learning cycle, its application to supervision including the need for each element, the more able they are to use these processes to achieve better outcomes. Practitioners find it helpful to understand how they learn (which part of the learning cycle they prefer to join) as well as why each element is needed.

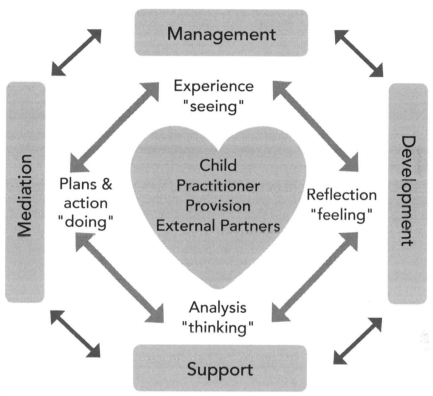

Figure 6.2: 4x4x4 Model of Supervision. Developed from Morrison T (2005) *Staff Supervision in Social Care.* **Brighton: Pavilion Publishing & Media**

Each provider will work out how frequently formal supervision happens. How the childcare is offered will affect the frequency of supervision. For example, many preschools, which operate in term time only, have an expectation for a formal supervision session to happen in each half term. For those providers open all year the expectation is monthly. Some practitioners, especially when they are new to the setting or inexperienced, may require more frequent supervision with a more directive stance. Perhaps supervision could be linked to the induction process and contribute to the performance appraisal about whether a practitioner is confirmed in their post (see Chapter 1 for a debate about what performance appraisal is and what belongs to supervision). Those who are experienced and have been well supported may manage with this frequency and should be capable of being more self-directive in their needs (see discussion in Chapter 4 about using coaching in authoritative supervisory practice). These timings would be an advisory minimal expectation of supervision.

Development of supervision policy using Appreciative Inquiry models of change

Appreciative Inquiry (AI) is a theory developed by Cooperrider and Srivastva (1987) which aims to bring about change by building on what already works well. It has been adapted for research and organisational purposes (Martins, 2014). A good starting point is to ask questions about the current situation before changing anything. This is the basis of the AI approach; just asking the first question brings about change. AI is a phased model of engaging a range of stakeholders in a process of change and therefore fits well with the challenges facing early years providers implementing changes of practice. Importantly the expectation is on collaboration from everyone with any interest in the issue, so that multiple perspectives are considered. AI also understands that how people and children relate to each other is significant.

Applying the ideas to supervision, what is appreciated about how supervision is working at present in the provision? The provider may start by asking a series of questions:

- How do supervisees and supervisors feel about supervision?

- How do parents feel about the quality of service or how their child is developing?

- How do parents feel about the information they receive from key workers?

It could be helpful to involve committee members, owners and the early years' advisers in the process of evaluating the current situation. Children may have a view about whether they like coming and the activities that are provided.

Noticing and paying attention to where there is consensus on what is working well is an important part of the AI model, paying attention to success builds confidence in the process of change. It is worth spending time gaining views about what is working well. Change has a tendency to focus on negative elements and valuing what is working well about the current situation genuinely engages practitioners in wanting to improve, as what they are already doing is appreciated.

Thinking point

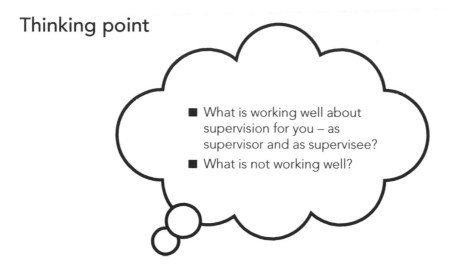

- What is working well about supervision for you – as supervisor and as supervisee?
- What is not working well?

Recognising that change is not going to happen for the sake of it will embolden people to say what they would like to see done differently and thereby move into the next phase. The first phase may have been done individually, for example through questionnaires; the next phase will probably involve joining together in some way to imagine a different way of doing things. It is important to identify who the key people are to begin the process of envisaging the future; there should ideally be representation from key stakeholders not just the managerial team. In this instance collective input generally produces better results.

For example once the end goal is identified, how will this setting know that supervision is working effectively? The key stakeholders need to find a way of deciding how to reach it. Originally Cooperrider and Srivastva (1987) used terms like 'dreaming', 'design' and 'discovery' for these parts of the process. Although those names can be off putting, it is useful occasionally to be reminded that dreaming of a future helps with designing the processes by which it is reached. What would it look like in this provision to have an effective supervision policy and culture, what steps do we need to get there? In every situation there are unintended consequences which is where the AI model offers flexibility, as the final process (discovery) recognises that while the design may envisage reaching a certain place (dream), there could be future unknown situations, which need to be taken into account and adjusted for. What ends up happening may differ from what seemed possible. The essential component in an AI model for change is recognising the fluidity with which human beings interact with their environment. This differs from linear experimental design models that expect outcomes that conform to the expectations identified at the start of the process.

Below is an audit tool which could be a useful starting point in identifying what the existing challenges are around supervision. Each provider will have made a start on these processes and this is once again a suggestion for discussion within the leadership team in each setting.

Thinking point

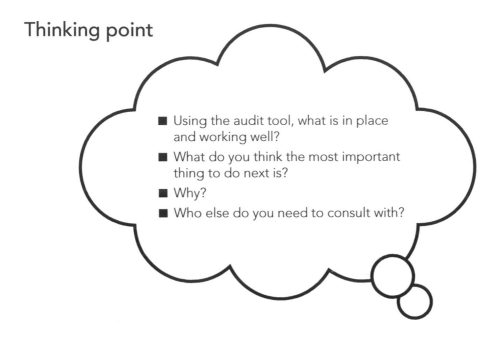

■ Using the audit tool, what is in place and working well?

■ What do you think the most important thing to do next is?

■ Why?

■ Who else do you need to consult with?

	Yes	No	In development	Action needed
As a management team are we clear about why supervision is important in the provision?				
Have we discussed the model and style of supervision that we wish to promote?				
Are we clear about the practical arrangements such as frequency and how supervision will be recorded?				
Is a written supervision policy in place?				

Is it clear how the supervision policy fits with other policies including safeguarding, staff appraisal and personal development plans?				
Have we identified the minimum training that supervisors should have before they start supervising?				
Is there a process in place for disseminating the supervision policy to both established and new practitioners?				
Is there training for supervisees on how to make the best use of supervision?				
What support is in place for supervisors? Are there robust supervision arrangements for them too?				
Are there plans for the ongoing development of supervisory skills?				
Do we have a system in place for evaluating the quality of supervision, including obtaining feedback from supervisees?				

Once the supervision policy has been worked out by the leadership team there is then a process of identifying how supervisors will be trained and supported in their role. Supervision training helps to build a culture that gets shared with other practitioners by supervisors being able to explain the purpose of supervision. Trained supervisors are better able to advise supervisees so that they prepare for and make good use of supervision. There then need to be processes which evaluate the quality and effectiveness of supervision, getting responses from supervisees and supervisors about the impact supervision is having on confidence and competence. By this point the expectation would be that supervision has become embedded within the everyday practice of the provision.

This chapter has reiterated the role of supervision in group childcare settings as a protective factor in keeping such settings safe for children. The link between supervision and safeguarding practice is an important one that managers and owners of provisions need to make sure their practitioners understand. Following on from this was a discussion about reinforcing the centrality of supervision by having a supervision policy. An audit tool of supervisory practice offered a framework within which to evaluate and develop the culture of supervision.

Final thoughts

Supervision is now expected to be in place in all early years settings and is a vital aspect of the service. Making supervision really effective can, however, be a challenge, and this guide has set out ideas and tools to help busy managers establish and maintain good supervision practices. As Chapter 6 identified, good supervision does not take place in isolation and will thrive in healthy settings where the focus is always on the needs of the children being cared for. It will also work best where those responsible for the quality of service delivery understand and promote supervision as a key aspect of their setting's work.

One important question remains – who sustains, develops and supervises the supervisors? This is an important question for any organisation but for early years settings it may need particular thought due to the variety of arrangements that may to be in place for delivering the service. It almost goes without saying that settings owned by large private companies will have very different management and governance arrangements to a small preschool run by a committee. These differences should not detract from the need to have in place arrangements for support and oversight of the work of those people who have responsibility for delivery of effective supervision.

Supervisors need to be adequately trained to do the job since untrained supervisors are unlikely to have the knowledge or confidence to deliver the type of effective supervision described in this guide. However, training alone is not enough. In order to sustain supervision beyond an initial training course, supervisors need the opportunity to stand back and reflect on their work, including the challenges of providing supervision to their staff team. How this is achieved may vary but must be an important question for all those responsible for the delivery of services to children in their early years.

Appendix

Checklist of functions

The support function checklist
The aims of the support function are:

- to validate the early years practitioner, both as a professional and as a person

- to create a safe climate for the early years practitioner to look at their practice and its impact on them as a person

- to clarify the boundaries between support, counselling, consultation and to clarify the limits of confidentiality in supervision

- to explore issues about discrimination in a safe setting

- to support early years practitioners who are subject to any form of abuse either from children or parents or from other early years practitioners, whether this be physical, psychological or discriminatory

- to monitor the overall health and emotional functioning of the early years practitioner, especially with regard to the effects of stress

- to debrief the early years practitioner and give them permission to talk about feelings, especially fear, anger, sadness, repulsion or helplessness

- to help the early years practitioner explore emotional blocks to the work

- to help the early years practitioner reflect on difficulties in peer relationships to assist the practitioner in resolving conflict

- to clarify when the early years practitioner should be advised to seek external counselling, and its relationship with the monitoring of performance.

The management function checklist
The aims of the management function are to ensure:

- the early years practitioner understands their role and responsibilities

- the early years practitioner is clear as to the limits and use of their own role, that of the setting and the role of the statutory authority

- the purpose of the supervision is clear

- the early years practitioner is given an appropriate workload

- time management expectations of the early years practitioner are clear and checked

- the early years practitioner acts as a positive member of the team

- the early years practitioner understands the functions of other agencies and relates appropriately to them

- the early years practitioner receives regular formal appraisal

- the overall quality of the early years practitioner's performance is measured

- the policies and procedures of the provision are understood and followed

- work is reviewed regularly in accordance with the provision and legal requirements

- action plans are formulated and carried out within the expectations of the provision and statutory responsibilities

- the basis of decisions and professional judgements are clear to you and the early years practitioner and written explicitly in the child's or practitioner's records

- records are maintained according to the provision's policies

- the early years practitioner knows when the supervisor expects to be consulted.

The development function checklist

The aims of this function are to assist the development of:

- the early years practitioner's professional competence

- an appreciation and assessment of the early years practitioner's knowledge base, skills and individual contribution to the provision

- an understanding of the early years practitioner's value base in relation to race, gender, religion, disability etc. and its impact on their work

- an understanding of the early years practitioner's preferred learning style and barriers to learning

- an assessment of the early years practitioner's training and development needs and how they can be met

- the early years practitioner's capacity to set professional goals

- access to professional consultation in areas outside the supervisor's knowledge/experience

- the early years practitioner's ability to reflect on his/her work and interaction with children, parents, peers and other agencies

- regular and constructive feedback to the early years practitioner on all aspects of their performance

- the early years practitioner's ability to generalise learning and to increase their commitment and capacity to ongoing professional development

- the early years practitioner's capacity for self-appraisal, and the ability to learn constructively from significant experiences or difficulties

- a relationship in which the early years practitioner provides constructive feedback to the supervisor and both can learn.

The mediation function checklist

The aims of the mediation function are to:

- negotiate and clarify the provision's remit

- brief management/committees about resource deficits or implications

- allocate resources in the most efficient way

- represent early years practitioners' needs to higher management/owners/committees

- initiate, clarify or contribute to policy formulation

- consult and brief early years practitioners about developments or information about the provision

- mediate or advocate between early years practitioners, within the provision, or with outside agencies

- represent or accompany early years practitioners in work with other agencies e.g. child protection case conferences

- involve early years practitioners in decision making

- deal sensitively, but clearly, with complaints about early years practitioners

- assist and coach early years practitioners, where appropriate, through complaints procedures.

References

Adams R & Mason R (2015) Free childcare: nurseries warn Cameron's pledge may cost parents more. *The Guardian* **1 June**.

Birmingham Safeguarding Children Board (2012) *Under Chapter VIII 'Working Together to Safeguard Children' in respect of the Serious Injury of Case No.2010-11/3* [online]. Available at: http://www.lscbbirmingham.org.uk/images/stories/downloads/executive-summaries/Published_Overview_Report.pdf (accessed April 2016).

Cain S (2011) *Quiet: The power of introverts in a world that can't stop talking*. London: Penguin.

Cooperrider D & Srivastva S (1987) Appreciative inquiry in organizational life. *Research in Organizational Change and Development* **1** 129–169.

Davys A & Beddoe L (2010) *Best Practice in Professional Supervision: A guide for the helping professions*. London: JKP.

Department for Education (2014) *Statutory Framework for the Early Years Foundation Stage* [online]. Available at: https://www.gov.uk/government/uploads/system/uploads/attachment_data/file/335504/EYFS_framework_from_1_September_2014__with_clarification_note.pdf (accessed April 2016).

Department for Education (2015) *Working Together to Safeguard Children. A guide to inter-agency working to safeguard and promote the welfare of children* [online] London: Department for Education. Available at: https://www.gov.uk/government/uploads/system/uploads/attachment_data/file/419595/Working_Together_to_Safeguard_Children.pdf (accessed April 2016)

Downey M (2003) *Effective Coaching: Lessons from the Coach's coach* (2nd edition). London: Engage Learning.

Erooga M (2012) *Creating Safer Organisations: Practical steps to prevent the abuse of children by those working with them*. Chichester: Wiley.

French JPR & Raven BN (1959) The bases of social power. In: D Cartwright (Ed.) *Studies in Social Power* (pp150-167). Ann Arbor, MI: Institute for Social Research.

Gast L & Patmore A (2012) *Mastering Approaches to Diversity in Social Work* London: JKP.

Gerhardt S (2004) *Why Love Matters: How affection shapes a baby's brain*. Hove: Routledge.

Goleman D (1995) *Emotional Intelligence: Why it can matter more than IQ*. London: Bloomsbury.

Green J (2012) Avoiding and managing allegations against staff. In: M Erooga (Ed.) *Creating Safer Organisations: Practical steps to prevent the abuse of children by those working with them*. Chichester: Wiley.

Hay J (1995) *Transformational Mentoring: Creating developmental alliances for changing organisational culture*. New York: McGraw Hill Education.

Kolb D (1988) *Experience as the Source of Learning and Development*. London: Prentice Hall.

Lambley S, Marrable T & Lawson H (2013) *Practice Enquiry Into Supervision In A Variety Of Adult Care Settings Where There Are Health And Social Care Practitioners Working Together*. Project Report. Social Care Institute for Excellence.

Marbina L, Church A & Tayler C (2010) *Victorian Early Years Learning and Development Framework Evidence Paper. Practice Principle 8: Reflective Practice* [online] Department of Education and Early Childhood Development. Available at: https://www.eduweb.vic.gov.au/edulibrary/public/earlylearning/evi-refprac.pdf (accessed April 2016).

Martins C (2014) *Appreciative Inquiry in Child Protection: Identifying and promoting good practice and creating a learning culture: practice tool*. Devon: Research in Practice.

Morrison T (2005) *Staff Supervision in Social Care*. Brighton: Pavilion Publishing & Media.

Morrison T (2007) Emotional intelligence, emotion and social work: context, characteristics, complications and contribution. *British Journal of Social Work* **37** (2) 245–263.

Nutbrown C (2012) *Foundations for Quality: The independent review of early education and childcare qualifications* [online]. London: Department for Education. Available at: https://www.gov.uk/government/uploads/system/uploads/attachment_data/file/175463/Nutbrown-Review.pdf (accessed April 2016).

Plymouth Safeguarding Children Board (2010) *Serious Case Review Overview Report Executive Summary in Respect of Nursery Z* [online]. Available at: http://www.plymouth.gov.uk/serious_case_review_nursery_z.pdf (accessed April 2016).

Sunderland M (2007) *What Every Parent Needs To Know*. London: Dorling Kindersley.

Wonnacott J (2012) *Mastering Social Work Supervision*. London: JKP.

Wonnacott J (2013) Keeping children safe in nurseries: a focus on culture and context. *Journal of Sexual Aggression* **19** (1) 32–45.

Wonnacott J (2014) *Developing and Supporting Effective Staff Supervision*. Brighton: Pavilion Publishing & Media.

Further resources from Pavilion

Bostock L (2016) *Interprofessional Staff Supervision in Adult Health and Social Care Services: Volume 1, 2016*
This annual volume looks at different models of supervision within adult services, addressing a gap in research and practice about what works when supervising staff from across different professional backgrounds, including social work, nursing, health visiting, clinical psychology, community mental health and addiction services.
Available at: https://www.pavpub.com/interprofessional-staff-supervision-adult-health-social-care-volume-1/

Knapman J & Morrison T (1998) *Making the Most of Supervision in Health and Social Care: A self-development manual for supervisees*.
A support manual for supervisees in health and social care designed to help supervisees understand the process of clinical supervision sessions.
Available at: https://www.pavpub.com/making-the-most-of-supervision-in-health-andsocial-care/

Morrison T (2010) *Staff Supervision in Social Care*.
In its 3rd edition this bestselling guide brings essential, newly-developed material, while retaining core material covering the fundamentals of good supervision.
Available at: https://www.pavpub.com/staff-supervision-in-social-care/

Morrison T (2008) *Strength to Strength*.
A training tool for supervisors, trainers and student teachers to prepare supervisees for supervision.
Available at: https://www.pavpub.com/strength-to-strength/

Wonnacott J (2014) *Developing and Supporting Effective Staff Supervision Training Pack*.
A training pack and reader focusing on training supervisors to deliver one-to-one supervision for those working with vulnerable children, adults and their families. Its flexible structure enables trainers to design their own bespoke training programmes.
Available at: https://www.pavpub.com/developing-and-supporting-effective-staffsupervision-training-pack/

Wallbank S (2016) *The Restorative Resilience Model of Supervision: An organisational training manual for building resilience to workplace stress in health and social care professionals.*
A training resource based on the sustainable model of professional resilience, to be used in supervision, coaching and supportive sessions across clinical practices.
Available at: https://www.pavpub.com/restorative-resilience-model-ofsupervision-training-pack/

Wallbank S (2016) *The Restorative Resilience Model of Supervision: A reader exploring resilience to workplace stress in health and social care professionals.*
This resource allows an organisation to cascade the restorative resilience approach throughout their staff, initially 'training a trainer', who can then pass the knowledge on to any number of supervisors.
Available at: https://www.pavpub.com/restorative-resilience-model-ofsupervision-reader/